Confederate Commando and Fleet Surgeon

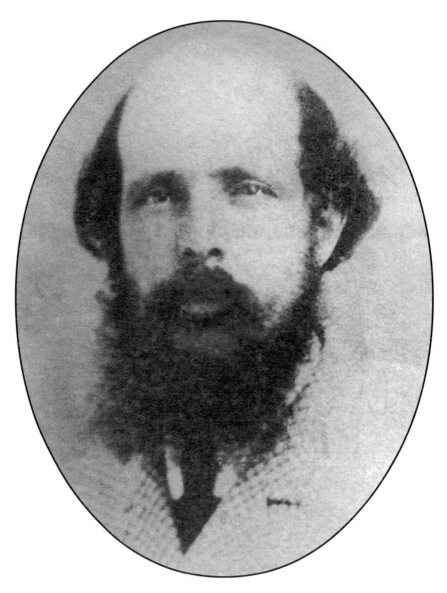

Dr. Daniel Burr Conrad, probably immediate postwar

Confederate Commando
and Fleet Surgeon
Dr. Daniel Burr Conrad

John W. Lynn

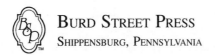

BURD STREET PRESS
SHIPPENSBURG, PENNSYLVANIA

This Burd Street Press publication
was printed by
Beidel Printing House, Inc.
63 West Burd Street
Shippensburg, PA 17257-0152 USA

The acid-free paper used in this book meets the guidelines for permanence and durability of the Committee on Production Guidelines for Book Longevity of the Council on Library Resources.

For a complete list of available publications
please write
Burd Street Press
Division of White Mane Publishing Company, Inc.
P.O. Box 152
Shippensburg, PA 17257-0152 USA

Library of Congress Cataloging-in-Publication Data

Lynn, John W. (John Worth), 1936-
    Confederate commando and fleet surgeon : Dr. Daniel Burr Conrad / John W. Lynn.
        p. cm.
    Includes bibliographical references and index.
    ISBN 1-57249-220-1 (alk. paper)
    1. Conrad, Daniel B. (Daniel Burr), 1831-1898. 2. Confederate States of America.
Navy--Surgeons--Biography. 3. Surgeons--Confederate States of America--Biography. 4.
United States----History--Civil War, 1861-1865--Medical care. 5. United
States--History--Civil War, 1861-1865--Naval operations. 6. United
States--History--Civil War, 1861-1865--Commando operations.

E625.C65 L95 2000
973.7'75'092--dc21
[B]   00-049417

Contents

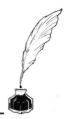

Illustrations

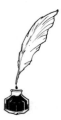

Foreword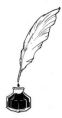

In the late 1980s, I was offered a large accumulation of letters and documents related to Dr. Daniel Burr Conrad of Winchester, Virginia. After reading them, I realized that I was being given a chance to buy a "piece of history." The more I read about his life, the more I realized how large a role Dr. Conrad had played in the Southern Confederacy. Conrad had been a Federal naval medical officer, a Confederate "commando," fleet surgeon at Mobile Bay and after the War Between the States, a pioneer in the infant science of modern mental health.

I searched the usual sources and circulated the word among some Civil War historians that I was interested in this particular man. I received several leads that, when followed, produced a bountiful crop of information. The following is a first harvest, because I am sure that others will come forward with new and important information.

Acknowledgements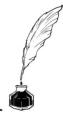

I wish to thank the following people who helped me write this book. Anne Bundy Lewis of Petersburg was instrumental in initiating my interest in Dr. Daniel Burr Conrad. I had an interesting and informative visit with Fielding Tyler of the Life-Saving Museum at Virginia Beach, Virginia. Bob Holcomb at the Confederate Naval Museum in Columbus, Georgia, and Michael J. Crawford, head of the Early History Branch of the Naval Historical Center in Washington, D.C., were particularly helpful in giving me leads for further exploration. John Emond of Washington, D.C., searched military records at the National Archives. Claudia Jew at the Mariners' Museum in Newport News, Virginia, was gracious enough to expedite several photographic copies of ships with which Conrad was affiliated. James Montgomery, the management information systems director at the archives of Central State Hospital, Petersburg, Virginia, and Richard D. Wills, management information systems director at the archives of Western State Hospital, Staunton, Virginia, gave me insights into the early history of the mental healthcare system in Virginia.

My thanks to Colonel Charles Waterhouse of Edison, New Jersey, for his permission to use his wonderful painting of the storming of the USS *Underwriter.*

Dr. David Powers of Winchester, Virginia, was kind enough to contribute to the completeness of this work. Mrs. Catherine A. Roller of Harrisonburg, Virginia, who is working on another branch of the Conrad family was generous with her help. I am very appreciative of the staff at the Warren Rifles Confederate Museum at Front Royal, Virginia, for their efforts to get a photograph of the uniform worn by Dr. William Davis.

My thanks to the staff of the Virginia Historical Society in Richmond, Virginia, and Rebecca A. Ebert, archives librarian, and staff at the Handley Regional Library in Winchester, Virginia.

Jodi L. Koste, archivist at Tompkins-McCaw Library at the Medical College of Virginia in Richmond, was helpful with my research of early Virginia doctors and medicine.

Paul DeHaan of Kalamazoo, Michigan, who collects Admiral Farragut and Battle of Mobile Bay memorabilia, graciously allowed me to use some of his unpublished material.

One of the two or three major contributors to my endeavor was Ben Ritter of Winchester, with his extensive collection of photographs. He was a citadel of knowledge about the Valley of Virginia.

My greatest appreciation goes to John A. Hedrick, great-grandson of Dr. Conrad. He responded to my inquiries that sometimes arose after I read some puzzling tidbit in a letter or document. Without his help, this work would have been impossible.

Chapter One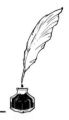

The Education of Dr. Daniel Burr Conrad, and His Service on Board the USS *Congress*

In May of 1861, young Dr. Daniel Burr Conrad returned home to Winchester, Virginia, from Boston, Massachusetts. For the previous seven years, Dr. Conrad had been an assistant US Navy surgeon on several gunboats cruising the Mediterranean and Caribbean Seas. Conrad's last cruise, before the Civil War, was aboard the USS *Niagara* which carried the first Japanese legation to visit the United States, back to Japan. On the *Niagara*'s arrival at Boston from Japan, its crew and 30 officers first learned of the great schism that had befallen this country. At Boston, while on board the *Niagara,* all but one of the Southern-born officers, after hearing of the firing on Fort Sumter, declined to take the required oath of allegiance. Nine of these officers were held in close confinement and eventually either were exchanged or escaped and fled south. Some of these nine officers became part of the initial core of officers in the Confederate navy who had had prior nautical training. A few of these nine joined Conrad in the Virginia navy which existed for a little over a month. After the dissolution of the Virginia navy, Conrad was assigned by the Confederate navy to the 2nd Virginia Volunteer Infantry as a passed assistant surgeon. Conrad joined many childhood friends on the train ride from Winchester to the imminent battle at Manassas Junction.

After serving at First Manassas, Conrad was assigned to New Orleans and later to the naval fortifications at Drewry's Bluff, south of Richmond. In 1864, Conrad accompanied the joint Confederate navy and Confederate marine operation of Commander J. Taylor Wood to New Bern, North Carolina, on the secret mission to capture the USS *Underwriter*. This small group of Confederate commandos boarded and captured the *Underwriter*, but due to the inability to generate steam quickly, this gunboat had to be set on fire and abandoned. Today, its hull can be seen at a very low tide in New Bern Bay.

Later, Dr. Conrad was assigned as fleet surgeon of the small fleet at Mobile Bay. Conrad lived on board the Confederate ironclad CSS *Tennessee*. He helped save Admiral Franklin Buchanan's leg when it was nearly amputated by an iron splinter caused by a cannonball ripping through a partially open gun port during the Battle of Mobile Bay on August 5, 1864. Dr. Conrad accompanied his patient as a prisoner of war to the Pensacola Naval Hospital. Conrad was exchanged after Admiral Buchanan was taken to Fort Lafayette, New York. Dr. Daniel Burr Conrad ranks in the forefront of most surgeons of the Civil War.

Daniel Burr Conrad was born on February 24, 1831, one of seven sons of Robert Young Conrad. The elder Conrad (1805-1875), a prominent lawyer in Winchester, Virginia, was a representative to the State Convention of 1861, which eventually passed the ordinance of secession. Daniel Burr Conrad's mother was Elizabeth Whiting Powell of Loudoun County. She, her husband, seven sons and two daughters lived in the large "Conrad House" at 12 North Cameron Street in Winchester. Young Daniel Conrad received most of his early education from the Winchester Academy where he graduated.

Daniel Conrad completed his undergraduate education at the University of Virginia which he attended from the fall of 1848 through the spring of 1850. For the 1848-1849 session, Conrad studied ancient language, modern language, and mathematics. During his sophomore year, he studied natural philosophy, mathematics, and chemistry.[1]

After finishing his two-year studies at the University of Virginia, young Conrad continued his education and graduated from the Winchester Medical College. This small local medical school with a faculty of approximately five members

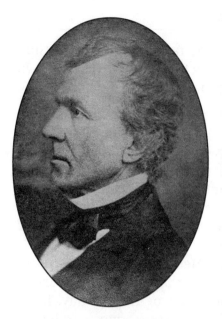

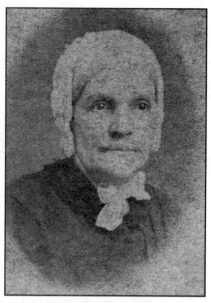

Robert Young Conrad,
father of Daniel Burr Conrad

Ben Ritter Collection

Elizabeth Whiting Conrad,
mother of Daniel Burr Conrad

Holmes Conrad Smith Collection, via Ben Ritter

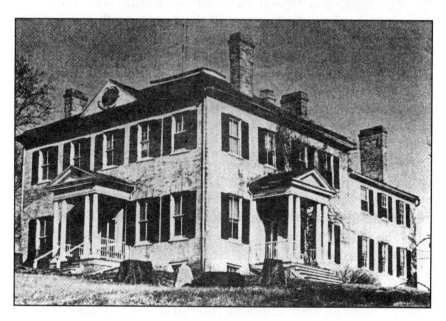

The Conrad Home
12 North Cameron Street, Winchester, Virginia

Winchester-Frederick County Historical Society, Archives

was founded by Dr. Hugh McGuire, father of Hunter McGuire, Stonewall Jackson's medical director. Hunter McGuire, who held the chair of anatomy, taught anatomy from 1856–1858.

The college building, a red brick structure with stone trimmings, contained a surgical amphitheatre with a large glass dome, two lecture halls, a dissecting room, chemical laboratory, museum, and offices....

In some respects the method of teaching in this school was a departure from that current in medical schools of that day. Instead of a curriculum crowded into four months with many lectures each day, the session of the Winchester Medical College was of eight months' duration, and the lectures were so arranged that there were only two or three a day. In this way time was afforded for dissection, parallel reading, and preparation for the succeeding day. Daily quizzes added to the thoroughness of the teaching, and a good chemical laboratory was maintained. Clinical demonstrations formed a large part of the teaching. There was no dearth of anatomical material, and many specimens were preserved for demonstration purposes. The custom of grave-robbing was, of course, in vogue, and the professor of anatomy was personally in charge of the students detailed for such nocturnal prowlings.[2]

After an earlier medical school had closed its door for several years, "...medical teaching was revived in Winchester in 1847, and under a new charter the Winchester Medical College opened its doors. The faculty now consisted of Hugh H. McGuire, Professor of Surgery...Daniel Conrad, Professor of Anatomy and Physiology."[3] Thus, Dr. Daniel Burr Conrad was taught in medical school by his uncle, Dr. Daniel Conrad, a prominent Winchester physician. This elder Dr. Conrad had graduated from this school in 1841 after writing his thesis on "Acute Gastritis."[4] The Winchester Medical College ceased to exist shortly after the beginning of the Civil War, after being burned by the invading army of General Nathaniel P. Banks

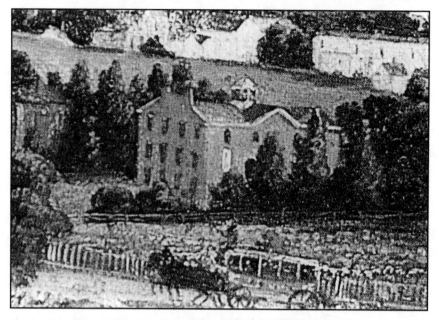

Winchester Medical College, before it was burned in 1862

This is where Daniel B. Conrad received his first medical education. This is a close-up of a print of a painting by Edward Beyer, *View of Winchester*, 1856.

Ben Ritter Collection

on May 16, 1862. It was rumored that it was burned by the Union troops because they discovered one of John Brown's son's skeleton at that medical facility.

Daniel Burr Conrad then took postgraduate medical studies at the University of Pennsylvania, Department of Medicine, in Philadelphia, where he received a doctor of medicine degree. "For years thirty or forty students had annually attended the sessions of the college."[5] Virginians had always made up a large percentage of the medical classes. "...up to 1860, there were 5,501 graduates in medicine from the University of Pennsylvania...1,749 from Virginia..."[6] On March 29, 1853, a memorandum of the Dean of Medicine stated, "the following having complied with the regulations of the schools and approved of by the Medical Faculty, are recommended to the Board of Trustees for the degree of Doctor of Medicine." On the list was Daniel B. Conrad of Virginia.

Prerequisites for graduation were that the candidate be 21 years of age and "must have applied himself to the study of medicine for three years, and been, during that time, the private pupil, for two years, of a respectable physician." In the "Catalogue of the Trustees, Officers, and Students," Daniel Conrad was listed as the "Preceptor" for his nephew. Daniel Burr Conrad graduated at the "Public Commencement" held on April 2, 1853; his thesis was on "Peritonitis."[7]

After completing his studies, Conrad returned to Winchester to open a private practice. Two diaries or daybooks, about two inches by three inches, written by Conrad are extant in the Library of Congress in Washington, D.C. On the flyleaf of one of these daybooks kept by Conrad, he mentioned that he rented an office from Washington Mosely on Saturday, June 3, and he boarded for $10 per month with the Miers, a local family. In his daybook, young Conrad listed some patients seen in May, June, and July, along with the services he rendered. In some cases, he noted whether his fee had been paid or not. He stayed in private practice for a little over one year.

Dr. Daniel Burr Conrad entered the U.S. Navy in 1854, after reporting for duty on June 15, to the Berkley Navy Yard. He received his appointment as assistant surgeon in the navy by the following letter:

> Navy Department
> September 25, 1854

Sir,

The President of the United States, having appointed you an Assistant Surgeon in the Navy from the 20th of September 1854, I have the pleasure to enclose herewith your Commission dated 22d. Ins't.

> I am, Respectfully
> Your obt. servt,
> J. C. Dobbin

Assistant Surgeon
Daniel B. Conrad,
U. S. Navy,
Winchester, Va.[8]

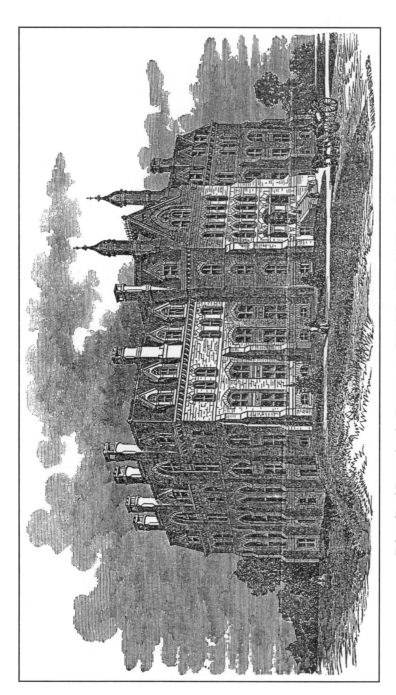

University of Pennsylvania, Department of Medicine, Philadelphia, Pennsylvania

Here Daniel B. Conrad received a medical degree.

USS *Congress*

This frigate was 179 feet long with a 47 feet 10 inches beam and depth of 22 feet 10 inches. On March 8, 1862, she had ten 8-inch smoothbores and forty 32-pounders. She was built by the U.S. Government and launched in 1841, at Kittery, Maine. She was lost on March 9, 1862, off Newport News Point, Virginia. During the battle of the *Merrimack* and the *Monitor*, "...she made directly for the USS *Cumberland* and the *Congress* retreated to shallow water. Unfortunately, she ran aground on a mudbank and was unable to maneuver against the Confederate warships. One by one her guns were dismounted by rebel shellfire until the white flag was finally run up, and a boat was sent to consummate the surrender. The *Congress*, however, was not allowed to survive, largely through the untimely resumption of firing from Federal shore batteries and snipers. Incensed that the Yankees should try and pick off his sailors, the Confederate commander of the Virginia ordered hot shot fired into the *Congress*, soon after which she became a blazing inferno. [It was at this time that Franklin Buchanan was shot through the thigh by a sniper.]

Eventually raised, the USS *Congress* was partially repaired but never of any real use again. She was later broken up and sold at the Norfolk Navy Yard."[9]

After some cursory training to be a naval officer, Conrad was assigned to the USS *Congress*, the fourth frigate sailing vessel to carry that name. On June 19, 1855, the *Congress* left New York with Conrad on board for a two and a half-year cruise around the Mediterranean Sea.

The *Congress* was the flagship for the Mediterranean Squadron composed of several ships including the steam frigate *Saranac*, the sloop *Constellation*, and the steam frigate *San Jacinto*. On board the *Congress* were:

Commodore Samuel L. Breese, commander in chief
Captain George A. Magruder, captain of the fleet

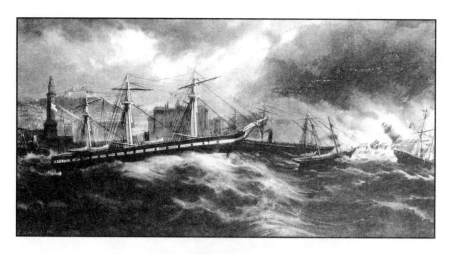

USS *Congress*

Frigate and flagship on which Conrad cruised the Mediterranean Sea from
June 1855 to January 1858

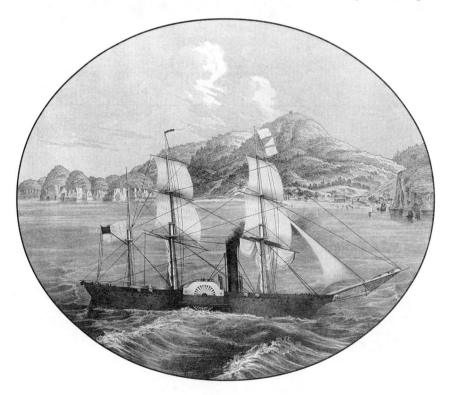

USS *Saranac*

Steam frigate that was part of the Mediterranean Squadron

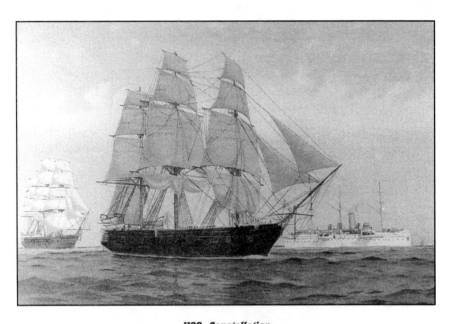

USS *Constellation*

Sloop that was part of the Mediterranean Squadron

Courtesy of the Mariners' Museum, Newport News, Virginia

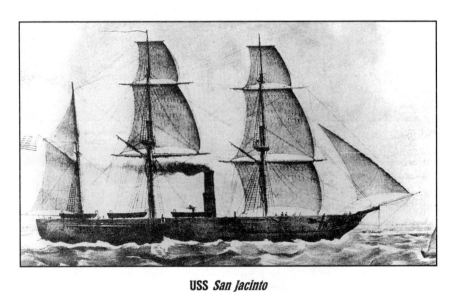

USS *San Jacinto*

Steam frigate that was part of the Mediterranean Squadron

Courtesy of the Mariners' Museum, Newport News, Virginia

Commander: Thomas T. Craven
Lieutenant: Samuel Marcy
Purser: James A. Semple
Fleet Surgeon: William Patton
Passed Assistant Surgeon: Charles Eversfield
Assistant Surgeon: Daniel Burr Conrad
Marine officer: Captain B. E. Brooke
Masters: B. P. Loyall
           William H. Ward
           E. P. McCrea[10]

Dr. Conrad told in his two small diaries or daybooks about interesting events at harbors visited by the various ships he served upon. Conrad described the first part of his cruise on board the *Congress* with the following passages from his diary:

JUNE—1855

Friday 15th—Reported, agreeable to orders, to Capt. Bearman at Brooklyn Navy Yard for duty on *Congress.*

Friday 22nd—First night ever slept on ship board.

JULY—1855

Monday 15th—6 P. M. Steam tug *Laviathan* towed us down along side of Staten Island—anchored—off next morning at 9.

Tuesday 16th—At 12, the ship anchored in Power Bay beyond the Narrows. "Practiced" in swimming, started at 9 A. M.

Wednesday 17th—Under sail, off the bar at 11:45 A. M. Pilot left us. Strong breeze springs up, then S. then E. My dreams whilst laboring under slight Gastritis were, of revelling in ice cold water swimming up to my lips, yet unable to taste it, going off in boat to icebergs, yet unable to break off any, every cooling drink I ever tasted were thought of, Mint julip, sherry cobbler, ice cream & yet all danced a maddening waltz around & around, yet never in my reach.

AUGUST—1855

Friday 3rd—270 knots these days. Off Azores or Western Islands, some 90 miles to the North—not in sight.

Saturday 4th—Making 10 knots, three hours ahead of time. Gained three hours daylight thus far.

Sunday 5th—Third Sunday at sea—840½ miles from Cape Spartell. Man died this evening at 3½.

Monday 6th—At 9 P. M., body enclosed in hammock with 32 lb. shot and dropped into the sea. Supposed, with this weight, the body will sink half a mile in upright position. Making 6 knots at noon. At this place we take tea at 6 P. M., corresponding to dinner hour in the States.

Tuesday 7th—Nothing of interest. Sea sick.

Wednesday 8th—Three weeks under weigh today. Heaviest seas yet. Gun deck wet fore and aft. Ship heavy sea. Heading directly down Spanish Main—East by South.

Thursday 9th—At 11 last night, the look out sang out "light on lee bow," the light house of Cape St. Vincent. This morning "Land Ho" after 22 days out. 10 sails in sight, most for the Straits. At noon, 130 miles off Cape Spartell. At night, wind & current carried down beyond mouth of Strait...[11]

Just after Daniel embarked on his cruise, his parents learned another son, Holmes, might be expelled from the Virginia Military Institute (VMI) in Lexington. Robert Young Conrad wrote the following letter to Daniel, in which the elder Conrad mentioned the possible expulsion of Holmes from VMI for acquiring too many demerits during his junior year.

Win.[chester] July 7th, 1855

My dear Dan,

Your letter was rec'd last night; & I have written today to Holmes requesting him to get your letters for Rome from Mr. Plunkett and forward them at once to your ship.

I am glad to hear that your associates are agreeable gentlemen; as it is a very important matter when you are to be in such close contact for so long a time: if possible it would be advisable to make friends even of the cockroaches:—with the bipeds, at least, it is easy and all important; and requires only a uniform, civil, good natured, yet some what reserved deportment, and the seizing of every opportunity to do a good turn, and sacrifice your own comfort in small matters to that of others. I do not fear but you will be popular with all classes; for I think your natural disposition is that way.

Your Mother & Kate arrived today whilst we were at dinner. Powell took the carriage for them on Thursday; & the heavy rains have kept them two days on the road. The younger set have been with me for a week or ten days; and with Salley's nice housekeeping & sweet temper, we have got along admirably. She is just now exulting in the gaiters you sent her from N. Y.—which fit exactly, and add nearly an inch to her stature. Do write to her, and when you get to Europe don't forget to pick up some pretty shells for her. The children all talk of you with much interest.

From Holmes, I have not heard a word, nor from Col. Smith about him. His trial examination was to take place on Tuesday week (Saturday June 30th), and Col. Smith had written to me that he considered his case hopeless, as he had 275 demerits, and 200 were fatal. But I wrote to the Col. and the Board a strong remonstrance against treating Holmes as an

ordinary & responsible being; as it would be like trying to keep a rocket in the straight path of a rifle
bullet; and I have some hope, as the Col. wrote me
that he would give Holmes every chance with the
Board, and I have heard no further, that they may
have pass him *ex gratia*.

No news here that would interest you. We are all
quite well—write again before you sail, and as often,
all the time, as you can. I will write again before you
leave; and as often as you will let me know where to
address you. Write to Holmes at Lexington—if only a
line—Yours aff'y

Rob. Y. Conrad[12]

Extant is a small, three-by-five inch Bible given to Holmes
by his mother when he went off as a freshman to VMI. On the
front flyleaf of the Bible is written, "To Holmes Conrad from
his Mother, Oct. 1852, VMI." A sketch of a VMI shako adorns
the page near this passage.[13]

After crossing the Atlantic Ocean, arriving at Cape Spartell
in Morocco, Dr. Conrad on board the *Congress* proceeded
through the Strait of Gibraltar and cruised the Mediterranean.
His ship visited the French ports of Marseilles and Toulon,
then the Italian ports of Genoa and Naples, then on to the
Greek port of Milo. Here, Conrad took a carriage to Athens
and was presented to the King and Queen of Greece. From
Greece, the *Congress* proceeded to Alexandria, back to Spezia,
Italy, and then on to Barcelona, Spain.

It was probably at this time that Conrad bought and sent
home a beautiful, highly polished slice of an olive tree from
the Mount of Olives. One side has printed: "D. B. Conrad, Ass't
Surgeon, U. S. Navy." and the Hebrew word for Jerusalem. On
the other side is printed: "U.S.S. Congress, 1855, Mount of
Olives."

The purpose of the squadron's cruise, though practicing
maneuvers, gunnery, and logistical support, appeared to have
been to promote international relations at the ports of call.

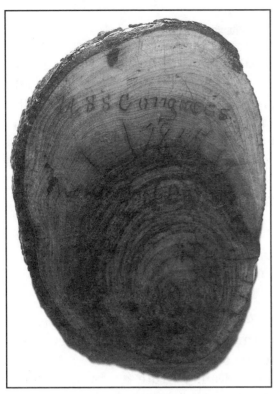

Polished slice of olive tree

Souvenir sent home by Dr. Conrad from Jerusalem while he was on the Mediterranean cruise aboard the *Congress*.

Author's Collection

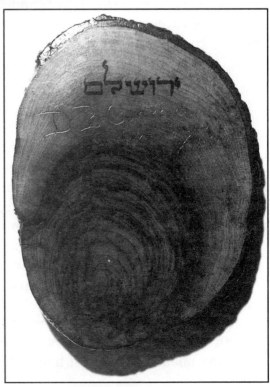

As the junior medical officer on board the flagship of the Mediterranean Squadron, it was Conrad's duty to go into each port visited and present his ship's "clean" Bill of Health. This was an affidavit that his ship and its crew were healthy and free of contagious diseases. Conrad would then receive a "pratique" which was permission for the ship's company to come ashore.

Conrad's last passage in this part of his diary reads:

November 1856

Saturday 8th—Calm fine wind, land in evening. In the track of the over land and steamed South for India.[14]

The final entry in this section of the journal in November of 1856 conveyed that Dr. Conrad mistakenly believed the USS *Congress* would steam "South for India."

On December 4, 1856, Daniel wrote his father, Robert Conrad, from Alexandria, Egypt, and described some of his adventures as he witnessed the bantering in the bazaars of Smyrna, Turkey, and his observations of the Crimean War.

> U. S. Ship *Congress*
> Alexandria, Egypt

My Dear Father,

We anchored here Sunday Evening (25th) ten days from Smyrna, where after a winter cruise in the archipelago, and within two days sail of Constantinople—our commander and unit went on board a steamer for the Crimea—ordering us to await him here—we had a stormy time coming through the archipelago—blowing a gale—raining so hard you could not see the ship's length ahead and islands all around us—there was very little sleeping that night—Our "Milo" pilot was much alarmed, for it so happened in that spot last winter a French line of battleships ran ashore and all hands lost, but ten men.—We were going about 10 miles an hour under reefed sail the

whole night.—When day broke, the celebrated island
of Patmos was astern and we in the open sea.—The
Orient disappoints you, nothing oriental or gorgeous
have I seen in either Smyrna or Alexandria, except
yesterday, the grand Barhams of nine tails airing his
ninety-nines,—some in carriages, some riding donkeys like men—short stirrups—their elbows resting
on their knees—all in their peculiar dress—head completely enveloped—only their eyes visible—loose trousers—and the whole person enveloped by a large
flowing robe of black silk—thin nails and eyelids
stained with "Henna"—the men squat in their bazaars
smoking—ride on donkeys smoking—walk smoking—I saw them sleeping with the pipe laying on the
mouth—and only take it out to wash and pray—this
latter operation, you know they perform at sunrise,
at mid-day and sunset, at which times the "muez-
zin" comes out on the balcony of the tall minaret
and summon the faithfull to prayer.—All business
ceases—they must go to the Mosque and kneel
around a high railing—I saw some kneeling in the
street at his summons—The bazaars of Smyrna are
superior to those of Alexandria,—both in point of
richness and being truly oriental.—You must imagine a very narrow street—dark, being completely
arched over—niches—nothing more or less in the side
of the house, about six feet deep, the same in height,
upon it.—The floor of which, the Turk sits, never
dreaming of rising to wait on you—with the eternal
pipe in mouth—if you want an article—you pick it
up, hold up before him and say "Piastre,"—the open
sesame—he holds up his fingers—half them or quarter them—you hold up yours just half the number of
times and then you generally come off cheated—their
religion allows them to cheat a frank, indeed, I believe it holds out some inducement to that end—And
this mode of valuation is after the manner of two

"rams."—I've seen them frequently meet in the street—touch it—the palms of their hands—and by way of being particularly affectionate, bring their foreheads together with decided impetus—then touch each others breasts with the finger—and take another butt—I can compare it to nothing else—this operation between two old men—you may imagine is rather laughable—I rode the other day to Pompey's Pillars and the canal through a flat sandy country—enclosed by hedges of date trees and cactus twelve feet high.— fields of sugar cane—gardens irrigated by small canals of a foot in breadth and depth—every other man, woman and child you meet blind from dust and heat—black gauze is worn over the eyes by strangers to ward off the dust—I thought of visiting Cairo and pyramids, but find the necessary expenses from here, amount to some sixty dollars, and cannot very readily spare that amount.

We left Athens on the 9th of November, whilst there I called on Miss Baldwin who you know is connected with Dr. Hill's schools.—She had received a letter from Winchester as you all were not mentioned, I had the negative news that you were all well. My last date from home was your letter dated 13th August. Where are the boys? Is Bob back at the University? Where is Holmes, and Sally is yet, I suppose at Mr [Yorks].—I have some pretty carved Lavas from Vesuveus for her—also some silk dressed for Mother and Kate—They will be sent home in the spring by the steamer *Savannah*—We probably go hence to Malta—if so, we will be there Xmas day which I can not realize is so near, for it has been one perpetual summer since leaving home.—Today, 2nd of December is very hot in the shade—we have all the summer vegetables on shore—though the consul tells me this is their winter.

Of the Crimean War—you gather more from the papers than I can tell—Tho' it is by no means ended, that Sebastopol is taken. The English officers whom I conversed with do not claim it—They lay the blame of their failure upon the officers, acknowledge with bad grace the superiority of the French whom they hate more than the Russians—Constantinople is the bone of contention now—You are amazed the French have occupied to the almost exclusion of the English and the general opinion here in Smyrna, Athens & Naples is that they will be combatants, instead of Allies yet—Are you amazed the English have occupied with several regiments Piraeus—without saying by your leave to King Otto—they have established a police there who control between it and Athens, by day and night—quarantine laws—also it is as much an English colony as Malta—The King and Queen have not been at Piraeus for more than a year—they declined paying us a visit and it being understood, they to get to us would have to pass through the army of occupation at Athens—You can hear the English revelry and from the Acropolis you can see the morning drill—with us, though at every post we anchor beside their men of war.—They never exchange a visit—their regiments now are composed of beadless boys though that is the case with the French—We have no idea of the power of the French unless you visit their navy yards at Toulon—we saw at anchor and in commission more "Men of War" than we have in our whole navy—at one time there were thirteen three deckers—each as large as the *Pennsylvania* at Norfolk at anchor. Did Mother receive my letter from Athens?—also one from Spegia, where I hope to be by the 1st of February, at least. And to find letter from you all.

The store ship, *Supply*, has just arrived here from Constantinople—you recollect, she brings camels to the "States"—Three or four have been presented by the various powers in the Lavant—The dromedary which is the "blooded" camel, corresponding to our blooded horse, is obtained here over—In Smyrna, the heavy built draught camel is bought—they average about $100.00—I often watched them being loaded on shore—kneeling down and refusing to rise if too heavily so—and in Smyrna, their long lines connected to each other by rope, passing through the narrow street—occupy it entirely—you have to get in the shops or store niches to let them pass. They seem to bear a particular hatred to the French or at least any one who wears brushes and dressing in a decent or becoming manner. Their bite scalps you, their kick demolishes.   December 4th

The *Savannah* has just anchored from Constantinople, we have not communicated as yet. Has on the overland mail from India, leaves tomorrow for England.—I shall not be able to give you an exact destination—write to me at Spegia.—My love to Dr. Corn. Smith—Aunt Harriet, cousin Ann and family. I'll write to Doctor David from Genoa—I understand a store ship will be sent shortly to Spegia with supplies—by it send me some more books—Harper's Magazines—we can buy nothing of that kind out here—Remember me to Cousin William & family.

Believe me, I am yours truly
D. B. Conrad

Dec. 4 1856[15]

In the following months, Conrad again visited Italy, then Carthage and Goletta in Tunis. Dr. Conrad wrote the following letter to his mother from the *Congress* describing an elegant dinner party he attended in Tunis.

Genoa, December 9th 1856
U. S. "Congress"
My last letter to you, My Dear Mother, was mailed in Toulon, since which I have received yours dated

September. We left Toulon on the 25th Oct., in a strong northwester. 'Twas for the first time a favourable wind, we made 180 miles before it ceased. Then we were becalmed for four days anchoring here on the 30th. We are now moored and secured near our old berth of last winter, I hope until next April. Tis the only place out here in which we feel at all at home. For here we find old faces and acquaintances of last winter. Many ladies who spoke English among the Genoese. We get the mail every week. This is by the ocean line to Southampton. But this winter there has been established a monthly line of steamers direct from New York to Genoa. We have now quite a respectable society of Americans here, the Commodore and ladies, Captain Wayman and family, Purser Semple and wife. She is a daughter of John Tyler of Va. and the wives of some half dozen other officers. This promises pleasantly especially talking English to ladies of which we do so little out here. We feel like foreigners when speaking it. And it actually sounds unnatural when proceeding from a lady. For you must know our only communication with them is through a horrid jumble of bad French. In my last letter I think I told you of my meeting with Mrs. Lizzie Bowzer, now Mrs. Knap in Tunis. Our visit was decidedly oriental. We called about 8 o'clock, were conducted into a gorgeously furnished apartment, found her seated on a divan and though not in keeping with everything around her, in European dress, we were kindly received and soon the party of eight or ten men luxuriously seated or rather half buried in the deep soft cushions of the seats lining the walls of the room. Dr. Heap clapped his hands and emerging from the outer darkness, some bearing in their hands, amber mouthed pipes with stems of twenty feet. Others, tiny cups of coffee flavoured with Attar of Rose. Men, some eight olive-coloured slaves, each done up in the most approved Moorish fashion. Can you imagine the luxury of the scene, sensing the fragrant *Latikia* tobacco, sipping coffee which you may imagine improved by the Attar, but in fact "twas all in my nose." Having that to as from a ship was luxury itself. Plenty of room and freedom of action, which our cushioned seats freely permitted, and of which the custom of the country permitting we freely availed ourselves, being waited on by an olive coloured face, crowned by a white turban, and terminating in a long black beard. The body enveloped in the indiscernible "*Burnouse.*" The voluminous britches terminating at the knees showing below a pair of yellow legs and the feet encased in yellow slippers. They stood, statue-like, outside the door awaiting the clap of your hands to fill your pipe or cup. To complete all, we spoke English.

Returning to the ship next evening, we chartered a little sail *Felucca*, such as are in use on the Nile and in it we sailed over the long lake between Tunis and the sea. The lake is beautiful, enclosed on all sides, except seaward by high barren, rugged mountains. The weather was just warm enough, being Wednesday 29th of October and we saw that rare sight, some thousand Flamingoes on the wing. They resemble pictures of those winged antediluvian serpents, such as geologists imagine, thin long neck and legs with intermediate crimson body, have that peculiar wave-like undulating movement when in motion. We have two Moslem boatmen, Mohammed and Ali, the former very rigid and exact in his religious observances. Ali was, I fear, somewhat of a backslider. There was a bottle of brandy in the boat to which he had free access, so by the time, we reached Goletta, in spite of his faith forbidding it, it was empty, and he was not drunk but "kingly glorious," singing, talking and insisting upon going on board with us.

Mohammed took all this very cooly, until he was paid, had tied up his boat, and said his prayers, probably as a sort of atonement for being so long in company and having had his boat defiled by unbelievers and Heretics. He then proceeded to "take care of" his partner, the glorious Ali, which institution consisted in the following. First knocking him down with an oar, then calling to his aid, some half dozen of swarthy black eyed "sons of the desert," they unwound his turban and binding him hand and foot, they dragged him off for purification, which does not consist merely in the free use of soap and water, but of a subsequent application of bamboos to bring about reaction of a healthy nature both mental and physical. Ali will doubltless long remember American officers.

Two or three days before leaving Tunis, a party of some eight of us were detailed to be presented to "The Bey." And such a dull disagreeable visit, I never wish again to participate in. We left the ship about 9 o'clock in the morning in an open boat. 'Twas raining in torrents and thus we sat huddled together for nearly an hour, as we lay nearly four miles off, you must bear in mind, we were in full dress, cocked hats, tight full dress coats, swords and epaulets. Landing at Galleta we found an Arab with a whip, presuming he was of the tribe of "Jehu," we followed him to his carriage. You know it requires rather a large vehicle to hold four men in ordinary array. Now add to each a cocked hat and sword. Then squeeze them into one intended for three and you have our condition. We drove through the rain for four miles over a rough sandy road to the Bey's country seat. 'Twas a long white and stoned building forming a square. We got out, entered through the archway, a paved court, three sides, covered with closely latticed windows, between which, the fluttering white robes of the inmates could be seen forming his harem. We passed on to the other side, through flocks of ducks, fancy pigeons, Shanghai chickens and a guard of ten Nubian soldiers arrayed in scarlet caps and pants, entered the anteroom and after resting in order to prepare ourselves for the coming event, we were ushered into the supreme presence of a short fat bearded old Moslem. He was gotten up in red tights, a scarlet fez cap, and green uniform coat and looking less like a Potentate than he did a Dutchman. There were some fifteen of his suite present, his Secretaries of State and Foreign Affairs on each hand, prompting his answers. He playing the parrot to perfection. Coffee with the nauseating accompaniment of Attar of Rose was handed around and then we had a "set to" in real oriental style, maneuvering, bullying and bragging. All which our Consul did in the most approved manner, assuring us it was "the custom of the country." For it seems that this old follower of Islamism had confiscated some property of Dr. Heap's and exacted tariff of the Consul, both which abuses he promised to rectify the next day. We then backed out, got aboard about 4 P.M. perfectly and thoroughly wet and disgusted. On reading this over I find Africa is the only theme, so I'll stop. Lest you may say like Dicken's girl that, "Africa is a beast and wish it were dead."

What numberless changes have taken place in Winchester according to your letters. I will have to begin life with Charley's acquaintances when I get home. Tell Sallie, we will go to parties together. My complements to Dr. Bob Baldwin and lady. Tell Tom Ricky, Miss Lizzie inquired particularly if he was married. I have written successively from Naples to Sallie, from Spegia to Father and from Toulon to youself. Have they all been received? I hope Mrs. Magill is better.

December 16

My last dates are those mentioned above. We have just heard of one of the new steamers being ordered out here either this winter or next spring.

My love to all and with you a Merry Xmas.

Believe Me My Dearest Mother Sincerely

Your Most Affectionate Son

D. B. Conrad

I send you the seed of Neopolitan melons. We bought some whilst in Naples in October and have seen yet not ripe. You see the houses festooned with them the whole winter ripening.[16]

Just a month before ending the cruise, Daniel wrote his mother another letter describing the tourist attractions in the city of Jerusalem. He vividly told of the pathetic inhabitants of the Lepers' Quarter and also told of tourist traps managed by charlatans to take advantage of the gullible.

U. S. S. Congress

Off Island of Caudia

October 5, 1857

The preceeding pages were written whilst in Jerusalem. The intervening two weeks have been idled away at Sea for we got under way an hour after we arrived and now that we are anchored here, watering and provisioning ship. The weather rendering candles supportable down in my room. I shall try, my Dearest Mother, to give you a journal of my trip. After "doing up" and I must say being thoroughly disgusted with the childish trumpery of the Holy Sepulchre. We started after breakfast the first morning to go around the city trails and see, what there can be no deception in, what man had let alone and stand in their natural state as they did when Christ was alive, the Valley of Jehoshaphat, the brook Kedron, Garden of Gethsemane, and the Mount of Olives. We ascended the Hill of Zion. On the top is the Armenian

Convent in which is shown the spot where St. James was beheaded. 'Tis kept as a holy shrine lit up with ever burning lamps in the night. To the right of this rises from the city wall, David's Tower. Further on is Zions gate now called David's gate. Just inside this a hundred yards off you see a row of low flat roofed mud hovels. Their low door ways front and separated about ten feet from the walls. This is the celebrated Lepers' Quarter, dirty and offensive beyond all description. There are said to be fifty of both sexes living here, isolated forever from the world. For no attempt is every made to cure them or better their sad lot, and once within their quarters, they are there forever. Here generation after generation are born, live and die. The wail of the just born infant mingling with the dying groan of the aged. I won't write you a description of the disease, all are deformed, some blind, some mutilated, trunks having lost part or all together the use of their legs and arms. When you approach them, they extend their ulcerous scaly arm, begging for alms. In all, the voice is like a hoarse bark of a dog, at first wheezy and husky, then subsiding to a low whine. They are supported entirely by charity—every one however poor throws them something—a bunch of grapes—a piece of bread or a few coppers. I saw one man apparently hale and healthy but who became infected by an accident and there he is to pass the remainder of his life. There are said to be some in these hovels who are so terribly deformed and maimed that from their birth to the day of their death, they are never seen by man. The disease does not appear in the very young. I saw one or two children seven or eight years old running about and playing on the house tops or in the narrow lane between the houses and the city wall. Going out of the city by Zion's gate, you first come to the tomb of David and here you have a fine view of the small village of Siloam and its famous pool, below is the valley of Jehoshaphat through it runs the brook Kedron rising from the valley and forming its father side is the Mount of Olives—lower down but in the same chain is the Mount of Offense. Now keeping close along the City Wall you descend the Mount of Zion, and then, ascend Mount Moriah—now you are at the eastern angle of the City Wall which encloses it, site of Solomon's Temple. The wall here is very high. At its base is formed of enormous blocks of greyish stone, beautifully and accurately hewn. They are supposed and with much probability to have been part of the Old Temple. For they are not only on the true site, but this is the only part of City Wall in which they appear. Most are thirty feet long by six in height. Rising high above the wall you see the dome of the great Mosque of Omar, in which no Christian dare set his foot, for this Mosque to the Moslem, next to that at Mecca, is the most sacred. 'Tis built over the central spot of the Old Temple, where rises a rock about twenty feet in height on which formally rested the Ark and the Covenant and on which the Moslem now shows the print of Mohammed's foot when he ascended to heaven. Thus this place is regarded by both Jew and Turk as peculiarly sacred to their respective religions, besides which projecting from the top of the southern wall, the Turk points out a round marble column which overhangs the great Valley of Jehoshaphat on which he says Mohammed will sit on the last great day to judge the faithful assembled at his feet and here at the same time, also you know the Jew believes the world will be assembled. Around this Eastern angle, you are at the base of the South Wall. Above you is Mohammed's column, to your left the gate called beautiful. This is now walled up and guarded day and night by Turkish soldiers because of an old prophesy which says that when the Turks are driven out of Jerusalem, through this gate, shall the Christian soldiers enter. Below you, you see the whole length of the great Valley of Jehoshaphat, traversed by the brook Kedron. To your left and on the opposite slope of the Valley at the very base of Mt. Olivet, you see eight olive trees enclosed by a high white wall. This is Gethsemane. To the left, a little way off is the subterranean Tomb of the Virgin Mary. To the right, on the same slope, the base of the mountain seems as if paved so numerous and so close together are the flat tomb stones of the Jews. Here are the tombs of their Fathers, and to this day are they buried here. This is the most peculiar cemetery, I ever saw; perfectly open and unenclosed, a barren sandy spot. Not a tree or even a blade of grass. Nothing in the world but thousands of oblong stones of nearly the same size laying flat along the slope of the mountain. Continuing along the South Wall you come to St. Stephens of the Sheep Gate. Following the road leading from this, you descend Mt. Moriah to the bottom of the Valley where you are then on the spot where Stephen was stoned. Then crossing the Brook, you begin the ascent of Mt. Olivet. Now nearly denuded and bare of its trees but crowned with the Church of the Ascension. To the left of the road, the first structure is, the Tomb of the Virgin Mary. Just across the road is the Garden of Gethsemane enclosed by high white stone walls. You are admitted by an Italian monk who gives you twigs from the sacred trees and pretends to point out the place where Jesus wept. A Bedouin Arab, who had followed us some distance, attempted to enter with us but was refused, the gate being shut on his face. We then toiled up the steep dusty road finding here and there a solitary tree until we reached the summit. We entered an enclosure, an Arab met us and first led us to the top of a high tower. Here I saw a scene which I can never forget. Towards the east, the horizon was formed by the towering deep blue Mountains of Moab, at their base lay the Dead Sea, emptying into it was the Jordan. Behind, were the rocky iron-like mountains of Judea. Before us was the entire city. You could see down into it, trace the circuit of the walls, the whole length of the Via Delorosa, and see the courtyard of the Mosque of Omar. The day was bright, brilliant and the atmosphere so clear that the outline of the Dead Sea could be distinctly traced. We remained on the top of the tower, exposed to the rays of the almost torrid sun. Perfectly entranced by the scene until the Turk neared and forced us down into the Church of the Ascension, a circular building with a vaulted roof, the sides perfectly bare but scribbled over with the names of a thousand travellers with a great show of awe, he led us to a rock projecting from the ground near the center of the building. On it was a depression like that of a man's foot. This was Christ's and to render it yet more sacriligious, he pointed to a hole near by made by his staff, perfectly disgusted—we took one look and left. Retraced our steps down the Mount across the brook Kedron and to our Hotel.

Leghorn Roads
October 30th

I've not mailed this to you, waiting until we arrived in a safe country for letters. We have been ordered home? Old news for you, I suppose. Was very sudden to us. We expect to leave Spegia by the 15th of November. Your letters, I've just received and was thankful for the good news. Kate's of the 5th of Sept. was the last. I hope Bob is better, the farm will suit him. I shall write from Spegia.

Believe me My Dearest Mother
Yours Very Truly
D. B. Conrad[17]

Later in 1858, after arriving back in Philadelphia from his Mediterranean cruise on January 13, Dr. Conrad was assigned to the USS *Plymouth*, an ordnance sloop, for a training cruise visiting various ports on the Gulf of Mexico. The top of each page of the ship's log states, "U. S. Practice Ship *Plymouth.*" This sloop-of-war was built by the Boston Naval Yard. The *Plymouth* had been assigned as a midshipmen training ship during the summers of 1855 and 1856. The *Plymouth*, now with Dr. Conrad on board, tested new ordnance under command of Commander John A. Dahlgren in 1858. The ship was again used as a training ship for midshipmen during the summer of 1859 and 1860 with Daniel Conrad still on board. He wrote this very interesting letter from the *Plymouth* to his mother.

"Plymouth"
Key West
July 14th

I've just written my all to Kate, my Dearest Mother, so you must not look for any thing lengthy. Our squadron is assembling slowly. There are eight at present in the harbour. The *Constellation* just from the Mediterranean has just arrived, Charles Fauntleroy on board. All are well. 'Tis a hard case that she should be ordered from here with all her old officers. None being allowed to leave for home. She goes with us to "San Juan." We leave Thursday and will probably arrive there about the 20th of August. It will be rather disagreeable, but we are ordered. The *Colorado* being disabled as a steamer and not being very effective under sail, she will probably go home to be repaired.

Lou is on board and may well I give him two boxes. One of jelly for you. Will you give some to my relations in Winchester and Martinsburg, just to them. I remember them, Cousins Ann & Millicent, Aunt Harriet & Nancy and others you choose. The cigars

are marked and boxes of the "best" for Father and
Uncle Holmes. The rest will be better when older,
and will keep. The jelly in this box, you had better
keep. It is from another part of Cuba. Only different,
no better. So much for this, one would think I intended going housekeeping. Send Sallie some boxes.

I received in Havana, two letters, Father's, and
Sallie's, and very welcome they were. The mail for
Central America leaves New York on the 5th and 15th
of each month & if you can write in time for the letters to arrive in New York, I may get them. I wrote to
Kate by the "Artic" which was ordered home and reserve your letter for the regular mail. I am unable to
surmise how long or even where else we may be ordered. Ned Tidball can give you earlier information.

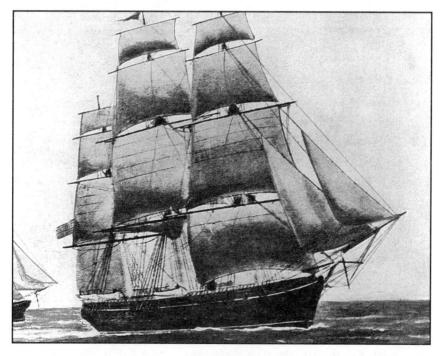

USS *Plymouth*

Ordnance sloop on which Conrad served in 1858, visiting ports in the
Caribbean Sea

Courtesy of the Mariners' Museum, Newport News, Virginia

It is thought Vanderbuilt, who has obtained from the Nicaraguan government, the right to contract a road across the isthmus. Will complete it in two months, then will be no further use for us.—July 21st—We sail tomorrow for Central America. I shall write you from there. My love to all.

Believe me my Dearest Mother

Yours Most Affectionately,

D. B. Conrad.

U. S. S. Plymouth

Care U. S. Consul

Aspearace, New Grenada[18]

Later that year, while still on the *Plymouth*, Conrad wrote to his mother:

"Plymouth"

At Sea

Off Belize

Nov. 13th

Although we have not anchored yet, my dearest Mother, I'll begin this letter hoping to announce our arrival either in Mobile Bay or off the mouth of the Mississippi tomorrow (Sunday) at least. Just as the wind favors, so will we anchor. We have today been fifteen days at sea with the minister, two ladies and three attaches. A doleful tale they will tell. Ten days past in a gale, for we've had three of them. Five days on ship's rations, for we all calculated on a ten days' passage. The ladies and attaches fifteen days seasick, for they have all a weakness in that line. The minister and all the party thoroughly and heartily disgusted, to an extent pitiful to behold with their fare, their accommodations and the magnificent ship sent to do him honor. For you must know the Department lead him to believe a steamer would be sent for him. We are now fifty-four miles from Mobile and fifty-eight from South West passage (for there are three) of the river. Capt. Dahlgren's intention is to go up to which ever of the cities we anchor off and telegraph our arrival to Washington asking for further orders. It is probable they may order us home. (Ned Tidball can tell you). It is possible we may be ordered to continue our cruise, probably back to Vera Cruz, for the city will certainly be surrounded by a besieging army. The minister speaks "ex cathedra." I am very anxious to hear from you all. Will you write, if only two lines, the day you receive this, to me at Pensacola Navy Yard. I may get it. If lost, well, we will certainly go there to get provisions and water, for we have run out and dependent on our orders, may remain there two weeks and then go to Havana.

Mobile Bay
Sunday Evening

Although it is Sunday, my dearest Mother, yet I must finish this as the letters are carried up to the city early tomorrow morning. We luckily got a wind and sent us into the Bay. Imagine the delight of the minister's party, especially their feelings of hunger. Please write me at Pensacola.

I shall write you before leaving here.
Believe Me
Your affectionate Son
D. B. Conrad[19]

Conrad's father wrote his son and told him the sad news of the passing of Daniel's brother, Bob. The younger Robert Y. Conrad was born in 1836, had graduated from the University of Virginia, and died November 14, 1858.

Winchester, Jan'y 13th, 1858

My Dear Dan,

I have just now taken your letter up to your Mother and heard it read and you may imagine how much rejoiced we all are to hear of your safe arrival,

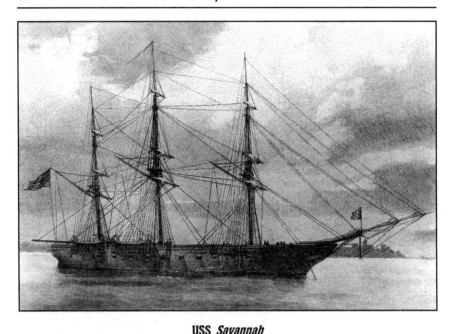

USS *Savannah*

Training ship and flagship of the Home Squadron
Courtesy of the Mariners' Museum, Newport News, Virginia

when we did not look for you until the latter part of February. You have been always in our thoughts and a familiar theme of our talk at home, so that I can hardly realize the fact that you have not been among us for nearly three years.

But, my dear son, there is one drawback to our delight at the prospect of meeting you again so soon. A sad affliction has happened in our family circle, which, while time has, as always, somewhat mitigated to us at home, must now fall in its original force upon you. I weep again with you. Your brother, Robert, is no more. His health was bad at the University last winter, and when he got home we thought it best for him to intermit one year and take charge of the farm. He grew worse then and came in, and after but a few days' sickness, died, on the 16th of November. He suffered but little pain and died from an effusion of water upon the brain. What the real disease was, could not well be determined—whether of the spine, as seemed to be indicated by complaint of his back for more than a year, and blood boils, or whether it was a rapid case of typhoid fever. He was developing the traits of a fine manly character, when thus suddenly taken from us. It was a terrible shock, unexpected to all of us around him, until a few hours before it was over us. Your poor Mother was yet more tired, being, at the time in Stafford Co. on a visit to Mrs. Brooke, and with great effort, traveled night and day only got home to see him buried. The rest of our family are well—Powell in Romney, and Holmes in Greenbriar, the others at home.

We all look for you anxiously—but do not wish you to leave until all your duties are performed. You will, of course, not think of resigning until we can talk the matter over.

Write again from Phil'a,

Affectionately Yours,

Rob. Y. Conrad

Doct. D. B. Conrad[20]

In 1859, Dr. Conrad was ordered to the USS *Savannah* for a training cruise in the Gulf of Mexico. He made no entry in his diary regarding his second cruise. The *Savannah* served as the flagship for the Home Squadron along the east coast of Mexico during the years of 1859 and 1860. Conrad conveyed to his mother how very thankful that he was to be able to get on this ship and take this cruise.

A few months later, Dan's father wrote a letter that told of being offered the chance to defend John Brown after his capture at Harpers Ferry.

Winchester, Nov. 11th, 1859

My dear Doctor,

We have received all of your letters, though I have not written to you at Vera Crus, did not reach you before you left there. Your determination to go on at once to Philadelphia was a great disappointment to us all, as we fully expected to see you at home, supposing you could rest yourself here for some days at least, before entering upon your studies. But it may turn out for the best. I do not wish in the least to weaken your impression as to necessity on your part for diligent and laborious study in preparation for your examination. On the contrary, I have felt some uneasiness myself, having heard that the examinations were more strict of late years, and fearing that you might be taken by surprise. But as you are aware of the necessity, and will therefore take care to prepare yourself, I no longer apprehend any danger of your not passing;—a contingency which would have much wider effect upon your future prospects than merely the fact of leaving the service. You will no doubt have seen Doctor H. McGuire in Philadelphia, and had the the benefit of his advice. From his acquaintance with members of the profession, he may also be of service to you, either directly or indirectly, in making favor with members of the examining board. If there are not yet detailed, get Edward Tidball to inform you as soon as he can of their names, and write to me or to Doctor McGuire who they are. If any are now in Philadelphia, cultivate their acquaintance; it will have the further effect of putting you at your ease when you come before them. I would also advise you to consult Hunter McGuire, and get him to aid you in your preparations. He partly from a natural adaptation, and in part from having been thrown by his father at once into the practice, is as good a surgeon now as probably anyone of his age, you can find and then you can depend upon his friendship and zeal to any proper extent. Let me know whenever you want any of your friends here. I suppose you would not allow me to caution you against allowing the Society and amusements of Philadelphia to take off your time or close close attention from your immediate business there. The subjects and methods of examination must be limited to some special fields of your science and you could probably ascertain by inquiry what they are. Whilst it would not do to run the risk of neglecting wholly any matter upon which, by possibility, you might be questioned, yet you might give your attention mainly to the most probable, and entirely to such as may certainly embrace all.

You might well be surprised of the foray at Harper's Ferry. Although it has now been several weeks past, during which we have heard little else talked of. I can hardly realize the fact as true. Old Brown sent for me on the first day of the court, offering a liberal fee to defend him. As he confessed and gloried in all the acts of crime, and would not agree even to the plea of insanity, I sent him word I could not take a fee in his case—(It would have been to defend the <u>crime</u>, not the <u>criminal</u>). but that he should have a fair legal trial, defended either by foreign counsel, whom he might select and write to, or, if they did not come, by myself or any other counsel directed by the court and without fee. He replied that he did not want a mock trial, & would have no counsel appointed by the court. I then went off to the Leesburg court where I had some cases to try:—and Misters Green & Botts, were at first appointed by the Court to defend him, and he easily in the trial repudiated them—as he would have done me. All have been tried fairly and condemned—except two, who are left to the tender mercies of Uncle Sam, with some view, (which will prove fallacious) of getting hold of some of the Northern mitigators. My own conviction is, that not only is the number of Northern sympathizers very

small and contemptible; but that neither Brown, nor
any of his band, were acting under the abolition fa-
naticism. He and his followers, were the remnant of
one of those lawless bands in Kansas, who for years
had been engaged in just such savage warfare. Finding their occupation gone, on the border, & driven
back into the states, their lawless habit of life, made
them unfit for civil life or pursuits, and drove them
into this desperate affair. Brown, Cook, Stevens, and
all are of this kind—merely desperate scoundrels,
ready for any such Kansas work, and not particular
on which side. One proof of this is in the fact that
one of his present party was actually engaged in Kansas, opposed to Brown, in one of the (so called) pro-
slavery bands.

We are a small household now, which makes us
more desirous to see you at home. Kate is in Richmond, with Laura Tucker, and seems to be enjoying
herself very much. Holmes is at the University, pro-
fessing the very best resolutions in the world, and,
as far as I can judge, pursuing his studies very dili-
gently. The little boys are all day at school, through
the week, and on Saturdays, in the woods & fields.
Kate's absence keeps away a good deal of the company she collects when at home, though Sally has
had several of her companions staying with her until the last week. We are all quite well, barring occa-
sional colds; and the town is quite healthy, and quiet
now. Charlestown is still kept in commotion, and will
be until after the hangings, which are timed (Browns)
for the 2nd and four others for the 16th December.
The military guards, intended for the double purpose of protecting the prisoners both from their
friends and enemies, number about fifty, night and
day and keep the town under military regime. Great
efforts will be made to have Cook—the worst of the

set—pardoned, or his punishment commuted. He has family connections of wealth and standing, who are trying their best, and have to some extent already succeeded, in distinguishing his case from the others. But they ought not, and I trust will, succeed in saving him from the gallows. The mischief is too great—and continuing—these Northern fools, the abolitionists are actively agitating—the politicians, on both sides, are using these subject for their own ends—and our negroes, in Jefferson & Clark, have been incited to burn, within the last week, several barns, and stockyards—among them, Doctor Wm. Stephensons.

Sally and your Mother will give you the news (if any) of the town. Write me soon.

Your Affectionate
Rob. Y. Conrad[21]

As the 1850s closed, Dr. Conrad would soon leave on his last voyage aboard a United States vessel. Japan had recently been visited by the expedition of Admiral Perry which was sent to try to show Japan the benefits of international commerce. Japan sent a legation to the United States to negotiate new treaties and guidelines. This legation was taken back aboard the USS *Niagara* and Conrad was the surgeon on this return trip.

Chapter Two
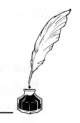

Dr. Conrad aboard the USS *Niagara* and the Cruise to Japan

In 1860 and 1861, Dr. Conrad ended his United States naval career as surgeon on board the USS *Niagara*, a steam frigate. This was a fairly new ship, having been launched by the New York Navy Yard on February 23, 1855. Conrad was on board the *Niagara* when she was ordered to carry Japan's first diplomatic mission to the United States from Washington to New York and then home to Japan.

For over two centuries Japan as a nation had been very reclusive. The country did not allow any commercial intercourse and all diplomatic contact was via a single Dutch ship that was allowed to visit Nagasaki once each year. Japan began to open up after the visit by the fleet of Commodore Matthew C. Perry to Jeddo Bay on July 8, 1853. [Jeddo, later known as Tokyo, was often spelled Yedo, Yeddo, and Jeddo.] A few years later Japan finally realizing the advantages of relations with the rest of the world, sent a diplomatic delegation to visit the United States.

Commodore Josiah Tattnall, returning from command of the East India Squadron aboard the USS *Powhatan*, brought the diplomatic representatives to San Francisco from Japan. The Japanese arrived at Washington, D.C., on the steamer *Philadelphia* from Norfolk on May 14 and were received at the navy yard by Commodore Franklin Buchanan.

The author has a copy of a song sheet that is titled "'*Powhatan*' Schottisch," composed for and respectfully dedicated to the officers attached to the US steam frigate

USS _Niagara_

Steam frigate on which Conrad ended his U.S. Navy career in April 1861

Courtesy of the Mariners' Museum, Newport News, Virginia

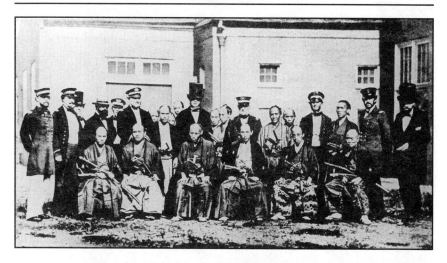

Japanese Delegation

This delegation was brought to this country in 1860 on the *Powhatan* and returned home on the *Niagara* with Dr. Conrad on board.

Charles Lee Lewis, *Admiral Franklin Buchanan*

Powhatan, during her cruise of 1857, '58, '59 and '60. The Japanese Embassy which recently visited the United States was conveyed on the US steam frigate *Powhatan*. The cover page has a beautiful tinted print of the *Powhatan*. The definition of a schottisch is a round dance resembling a polka. The schottisch was written by Edward R. Archer, US Navy, who would later be a Confederate agent at Tredegar Iron Works at Richmond.

Robert Y. Conrad wrote to one of his sons on June 5, [1859] that, "Dan has every prospect of a fine trip around the world. His ship is one of the finest afloat and Japan is one of the most interesting countries he could visit." He also says that "Dan hopes to see us before he sails but is doubtful...He sent Charlie a check for $50 for a pedestrian tour for his health."[1]

Captain William W. McKean was in command of the *Niagara*. The ship sailed, heading for Panama, on May 15, but due to the need for repair, the ship returned to dry dock on May 25. Conrad told about this aborted first attempt in the following letter.

U. S. S. Frigate Niagara
At Sea
Supposed to be 30 Miles off

Sandy Hook

Thurs. Night

Your surprise at receiving this, my Dear Father will but be greater than my own. When roused up at midnight some three nights ago to hear that the captain had called a consultation of all the naval officers and that they were debaiting [sic] the question whether we could safely proceed on our way, or had better put back without repair. It seems that as we were ordered by the Department "to fit out with all possible dispatch and proceed to sea on the 15th <u>at all hazards</u>," that the engines were not properly put in order. There was not time. Now we have one broken down engine perfectly useless, and all leaking six feet an hour. This is rather enormous, if you consider that the ship is 550 feet long and this length of water of variable width six feet deep. The propeller shaft was not well fitted with a circular rim of metal where it projects from the stern which fills up the orifice, prevents all leakage; yet allows of rotation. This parted and consequently have an enormous leak, fifteen feet below watermark. This could not be gotten at, at sea. So we will have

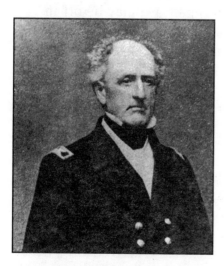

Captain Franklin Buchanan, USN

This photograph was taken just prior to the Civil War. Captain Buchanan on board the USS *Susquehanna* accompanied Commodore Perry on his expedition to Japan in 1852 and 1853.

Charles Lee Lewis,
Admiral Franklin Buchanan

to get into a dry dock, and have the sleeve of the shaft (so it is called) cast and fitted on, and one of the engines put in running order. We could not if we had proceeded fulfilled the orders, to make all possible dispatch and came up to the expectations, viz. "the Department expects you to be in Panama in sixty days." We have made up our minds to be timely reprimanded by an imbecile power. When their's was the fault. We were six hundred miles from land when we turned back. The ship is magnificent, sails twelve miles per hour and with steam we went fifteen. We had bad weather for one day. Though the men were not aware of it, when below deck. She is so immense that Atlantic waves do not move her much. Our quarters are very large and everything promised a pleasant cruise. What will be our destiny is only problematical, if ordered to repair, we may be off in two weeks. If ordered to await to convey the Japanese to Japan which we hope to do. We have just arrived and into the dry dock immediately. I shall write you again.

Yr. Obt. Srv't.

D. B. Conrad

Friday[2]

Conrad was the surgeon on the *Niagara* when it again left on June 30, to carry the Japanese delegation back to Japan by way of the Cape of Good Hope. The delegation consisted of 16 people. The first port the *Niagara* visited was Porto Grande, Cape Verde Islands. They arrived on July 16 and left two days later. Then he visited Sao Paulo-de-Loande (now Luanda), Angola; then Batavia (now Djakarta), Java; and Hong Kong. The frigate entered Jeddo (now Tokyo) Bay on November 8 to land their distinguished passengers. The log of the ship states that on November 21, 1860, it "received from Japanese government for use of the ship, 50 bags of rice, 5 cows, 30 pigs, a number of fowls, 15 bags of flour, 10 bags of beans, 10 bags peas, and a quantity of vegetables and eggs." The *Niagara* sailed for Hong Kong, leaving there on November 27, then to Aden, and Cape Town, South Africa. They were at anchor in the harbor of Cape Town from February 23 until their departure on March 9. Conrad arrived at Boston Harbor on April 23, 1861, and heard for the first time the grim news the hostilities had begun. Conrad and several other officers with Southern allegiances were asked to leave the ship. The *Niagara* was quickly resupplied and assigned for duty to help blockade the Southern ports and she arrived off Charleston, South Carolina, on May 10.

In the patriotic magazine *Blue and Gray* dated January 1895, Dr. Conrad wrote of his experiences upon his arrival back in this country from Japan. In the article titled "Reminiscences of Fort Warren—1861," Conrad related:

> Even at this late day we Southern-born officers of the U. S. Navy who happened to be attached to sea-going ships of war in either the African, East Indian, or Mediterranean squadrons in 1861 entertain very lively recollections of the manner in which we were received and welcomed home in the ports of New York and Boston. We truly had a hard time of it in resigning and getting South. In all cases—there were thirty-five of us—we were denounced in no measured terms and published in the daily papers as "traitors," and then imprisoned in either Fort Warren or Fort Hamilton for many long, weary months, in some instances running into a year. We suffered great pecuniary loss; our sea-pay, due us but not drawn from the purser (or paymaster now), in amounts from five hundred to one thousand dollars, was witheld from us.
>
> We of the *Niagara* heard whilst in the harbor of Hong Kong, late in 1860, that the election of a new President had aroused the attention of foreign nations and had excited the most bitter feelings between the

Northern and Southern States, following as it did the John Brown raid and other stirring incidents in the border States. Secession was threatened, and civil war was spoken of as not improbable. Thus the rumors ran in Hong Kong. Orders were soon received to return to the United States and proceed to Boston. On our arrival at Cape Town, in March, 1861, we heard that one Lincoln, a heretofore unknown Western man, had been elected by a plurality vote only; that the cotton States were consulting whether to secede before his inauguration. This was all we could hear or gather from the English papers. So when on April 12, 1861, we steamed up Nantasket Roads off Boston and were boarded by the pilot, who on being asked, 'What is the news in the United States?' replied in harsh, brattling tones, 'The United States have gone to hades, and they are hard at it fighting,' it was received in deep silence by all; caused us who had been in the service from ten to thirty years to ponder deeply, and even the volatile midshipman of fifteen years stopped and thought. What was the meaning of all this? Was the secession of some States the cause of this 'fighting'? Was there no other cause? How could this great nation be split up and sundered so suddenly? Were we destroyed? What was each of us to do? What was expected of us? Stunned and overwhelmed by this sudden catastrophe, we clustered into knots, asking, Which is the government? What side is ours? The pilot says that yesterday the *U.S.S. Pawnee*, with U. S. naval officers, burnt the Norfolk navy-yard and destroyed all the U. S. ships there, and that the day before Southern officers had threatened to destroy Fort Sumter, in South Carolina, which is defended by United States troops. We were all dazed by these seemingly irreconcilable facts. Who was who? and why were these acts of actual war done?

Nothing more could be gotten out of the pilot, so the next morning we anchored off Long Wharf; there we were immediately boarded by a very mysterious commander of the navy, who announced himself as a special government officer, charged with written instructions for the captain of the *Niagara*. A new oath (the ironclad) was to be administered to all officers. Those refusing it were to be detained on board and then sent to Fort Warren (in sight some miles away) and there kept as prisoners of war. This to be done instantly, he would await the result. He would hold no converse with any Southern officer on board, though many were old shipmates.

Kind-hearted old Captain McKean, of the *Niagara*, had all officers summoned into his cabin, had the new oath read and his instructions, tears coursing down the kind old man's cheeks. Nine of us out of thirty refused to take the oath. Then we awaited our fate. That evening the vessel was ordered to blockade Pensacola. As she was to sail the next morning, we could no longer remain on board. Fort Warren was reported without officers, and not yet ready for any occupants. So the quandary was relieved by Governor Andrew, who kindly offered to send us all to the penitentiary, and safely keep us there until the fort was prepared, his guards to be on board ship for us by sun-down. To this indignity Captain McKean firmly refused to be a part. Without his knowledge we left the ship in our boats. We had been told that our only place of safety was the navy-yard. In rowing thither we passed a vast assemblage of men on Long Wharf, prepared with halters and ropes to receive the "traitors," our names having been given in the morning papers, which also advised the mob to so receive us on landing. Avoiding this undesirable reception committee, we pulled into the basin of the navy-yard, where we were warmly welcomed by many naval officers, who sympathized with us in our forlorn condition. They kept us and protected us until night, when some escaped by way of Canada. The rest of us attempted the next morning to escape by train to the West and New York, but were arrested in the cars by Governor Andrew's guards, and were taken to the mayor's office for safe-keeping until the penitentiary vans could be brought there. The mayor declined positively to be a party to placing us in the penitentiary, and sent us under guard to the commandant of the navy-yard, where we were placed on board the receiving ship, but were allowed to go about on our parole not to attempt to escape. There we remained from ten days to three weeks, when every morning, on reporting at the commandant's office, we were one by one dismissed from the navy and taken over to Fort Warren, where we remained, most of us, until July, 1862, when we were exchanged for officers captured in the battles around Richmond.

The *Richmond* arriving some weeks later, and anchoring in the Narrows of New York harbor, was boarded by this same special government officer. He read the proclamation of President Lincoln calling for seventy-five thousand troops. The ironclad oath was offered, but was refused by some ten officers. These were ordered immediately into a tug-boat, already in waiting, and by sunset they were snugly and securely lodged in the casemates of Fort Hamilton; thence in a few days transferred to us in Fort Warren, where we all met again, having parted many months before, off Hong Kong. Here we exchanged news and encouraged each other, slept and lived in the damp casemates, permitted to exercise at certain hours, and occasionally to walk on the parapet. We were at times permitted to receive letters, all previously opened and read. No friends were ever allowed to visit us. Our only news was through the Northern press, and so we existed day by day, chafing terribly, when active life and active service and actual war was raging so terribly all around us and in our own homes. Some few of us got special exchanges for members of Congress and citizens captured at Bull Run or elsewhere, but finally all of us, after the seven days fight around Richmond were exchanged for officers captured in those actions. We were sent to Fortress Monroe, thence by flag of truce to City Point, and no one can tell how full of joy we were when warmly and kindly received by our Southern friends in Richmond."[3]

Conrad related the cruise of the *Niagara* in his diary by the following passages:

THIS IS THE CRUISE OF U. S. STEAM FRIGATE *NIAGARA*
May 15th—for Panama, Returned 25th
Sailed again for Jeddo June 30th
With Japanese Embassy, 16 in number on board—
On 16th of July, anchored at Porto Grande
Left 18th—On 6th August, at St. Paul de Loando left 15th.
Embassy landed at Jeddo Saturday 10th November.

MAY 1860-61

MAY—1860

Sailed in U. S. S. Frigate *Niagara* from New York, Tuesday, May 15th 1860. anchored off Battery—went ashore—payed visit near Central Park until 1 P. M.

Wednesday 16th—Remained on board

Thursday 17th—Got under way, went down off Fort Hamilton. Bad rainy weather. Got letter from Mother dated 15th May.

Saturday 19th—At 3 P. M. steamed out, at 7 outside made all sails.

Sunday 20th—Fine S. W. wind going 12—13 knots. Sail and steam.

Monday 21st—Fine weather. Rolled badly at night. Carried away main topmast, at night all sails folded. Under steam way at 7 to 8 knots.

Tuesday 22nd—At evening, the Captain called a consultation of the officers in the Wardroom on a report made by our Chief Engineer Williamson that the sleeve of the propeller shaft had parted and the ship leaking badly, four feet an hour. They determined to return to the U. S. The ship was headed to the west ——— to our surprise the next morning.

Friday 25th—Morning early, passed Sandy Hook at 11 A. M. Anchored off to the Battery. The Dunkey Pumps going since Tuesday to free us.

Saturday 26th—Went ashore. In evening, found this ship had joined to the gang. I on board the *Roanoke* with Lieut. Powell. Paid a visit to D. that A. M.

Sunday 27th—Last day near by Desolution, took men to hospital

Monday 28th—On board all day—landed Allegany dock.

Tuesday 29th—Paid a visit ashore

Wednesday 30th ——— Papers we are to carry the Japanese to Japan by Cape Good Hope.

JUNE—1860

Monday 25th—Ball to Embassy—up till 4$^1/_2$

Wednesday 27th—Steamed down off the Battery.

Thursday 28th—Ashore for last time. *Great Eastern* came, in went down with Miss D. to see her, came off.

Friday 29th—All day waiting for Harriet. Came to bring the Embassy on board, they came at last at 4 P. M. Manned yards, saluted all in full dress. Grand collection of New York rowdies in (Common Council) in ward room. No one allowed to leave ship.

Saturday 30th—At 1 P. M., under way, passed *Adriatic.* Coming in good weather

JULY—1860

Sunday 1st—General ——— church. Japs settling down.

Monday 2nd—good weather, wind ahead.

Monday 16th—Anchored at 8 P. M. in Porto Grande one of Cape De Verdes. Sent letter home to Father.

Wednesday 18th—After filling in coal at 5 this morning, got off. Good Trade, N. E. weather.

Wednesday 25th—In 10 degrees North got S. East winds, dead ahead. Have had them for past 6 days.

Friday 27th—Am now short of coal and water, have been under steam every day. Heading for Princess Islands, expecting calms and southerly current.

Sunday 29th—This evening at 8 P. M., crossed the Equator. Have S. East trader from 10 degrees north.

AUGUST—1860

Wednesday 1st—Passed Ilse of Aurbona. Calms and light S. E. Traders, heading direct for St. Pauls Loaudo.

Thursday 2nd—At midnight found the coal short only 20 tons, stopped steaming, under sail. Put on Quart of water.

Friday 3rd—Coast of Africa in sight, just off Mouth of Congo. Going $3^1/_2$ to 4 knots. 175 miles from

Sound, made 25 miles. Wind light from S. E. Heavy weather. On very short allowance of water, damp heavy weather. At 6 P. M., anchored by Ridge, until 3 A. M.

Saturday 4th—Dark, boggy weather—Light wind S. W., current one knot an hour from Southward, going 3 knots driving 1 per hour at 10 P. M. going $3^1/_2$ S. E. by S.

Sunday 5th—on short allowance of water, dead calm, drifting to North. At 10 P. M. lowered sails, got up steam at 12, going 4 knots.

Monday 6th—Going 4 to 6 under steam. At 1, sighted land. Making for Loaudo. At 5 sighted the ships at anchor. At $6^1/_2$ anchored. Loyall, Tattnall & Foster from the *Constellation* came on board, had general rejoicing. 3 ships in.

Tuesday 7th—Dined on board *Constellation.* The ship got under way, went to surprise Colonel Ripley & I went ashore first time since 28 of June. Saw the Negro town.

Friday 10th—*Constellation* came back have seen *Marion, Mystic, Mohican, Niagara* and *Constellation,* 3 English gunboats, 3 Portugese and 10 merchant sail.

Sunday 12th—*San Jacinto* came in. *Marian* ordered home. Went ashore with Loyall, walked out to well 80 feet deep, 30 diameter, saw cone like trees, 20 in height, 47 around at base, 2 at top. Bears a gourd fruit purgative.

Monday 13th—*Marion* sailed for U. S. Sent two letters by her to Mother & [illegible]. The weather thus far on $8^1/_2$ South is very pleasant. Cloudy in morning, clears up at 10. Sun shines during day. Observed during past four days 8 or 10 spots on sun evident at sunset. Three slave vessels have been taken one by *Mohican* with 900, one by *San Jacinto* with 620, one by *Sumpter* with $10,000 on board. Slaves s*ent to* Monrovia. Ships & officers taken to U. S. by foreign crew.

Tuesday 14th—On shore in morning, saw embarkation of old Governor. Had dinner party in evening on board the *Constellation* [with] Loyall.

Wednesday 15th—Great hurry this morning. Every one lost his wash clothes. Under steam at 2 P. M. L & J & B on board. At 4 P. M., up anchor and off. Outside, the Flag signalized "Assist the Boat." After laying to for an hour, man with some wines came on board.

Friday 17th—Smooth sea, perfectly calm. going 7 knots, burning 33 tons a day, coasting some 25 miles off, no land in sight.

Saturday 18th—Cloudy and calm, in evening, old rainy wind, thermometer at 60 degrees at 13 degrees South. Coasting along, land not visible, wind ahead.

Tuesday 21st—Cool weather at 22 degrees; 65 degrees at night, rain & cold. No fair wind yet. Dead ahead. No sail set fine. Bay Loando. Sea has been very smooth & calm. Swift wind. On 20th, were followed by numbers of Sea Fowl, Cape Pidgeon, gamets, & c.

Friday 24th—Blowing fresh from S. East wind.

Saturday 25th—Under Latitude 30 degrees 33 minutes. Steam at night Saturday. Cleared off beautifully.

Sunday 26th—No wind, cloudy. Just off pitch of Cape at 2 P. M. Wind from N. E. Under Royall & [illegible] 8 knots. Fishing for Albatross & Cape Pidgeons.

Monday 27th—Beautiful, clear, calm day. At sundown, strong breeze from S. E. going $10^1/_2$ to 11 knots. Close hauled.

Tuesday 28th—Heavy gale blowing S. E., dark rainy. Ship behaving beautiful. Very heavy seas, caught 3 albatross, $10^1/_2$ feet wing to wing. In evening, wind changed to N. East, cleared off, in latitude 38 South.

Wednesday 29th—Fine wind N. E. by N. to N. by West. Going 10 to $12^1/_2$ knots, wind on quarter, very heavy sea.

Friday 31st—Calm & clear, very heavy swells at night.

SEPTEMBER—1860

September 1st, 2nd & 3rd—Blowing hard gale. Sea very heavy. Ship wonderfully easy. On latitude 40 South 39 East. Very cold. Albatross are merciless, uncertain where to go to Mauritius or Batavia. Wind N. E. by E.

Tuesday 4th—S. E. gale with heavy sea, very cold, dark rainy. 42 degrees 30 minutes South at noon—moves ship to N. by E. at 6 P. M. taken back by S. W. wind, going 9 knots to Mauritius. First wind, sails not hauled. Should have steered for Java Head, (Batavia), bad night.

Wednesday 5th—Suddenly our course is changed for Batavia. We now are 42 degrees South; nothing but ship's rations.

Saturday 8th—Fine N.W. wind going E. by S. 10 Knots.

Thursday 13th—Caught albatross, affixed copper plate with Lat. & Long., name and let go.

Friday 14th—Cold day, sky bright. At 1 P. M., sighted New Amsterdam, high island.

Saturday 15th—Pleasant day, morning fine wind N. W. by N. In evening, rain squalls very heavy. Very cold.

Sunday 16th—Fine day, very cold. Number of albatross. In evening, cool and cloudy. Very dark.

Monday 17th—

Tuesday 18th—

Wednesday 19th—

Thursday 20th—

Friday 21st—Got up steam.

Saturday 22nd—

Sunday 23rd—Beautiful day, wind stopped, raining.

Monday 24th—The Traders, at last. Not from S. E., as hoped.

Tuesday 25th—Traders from E. by S., first at times.

Wednesday 26th—Traders from E. by S., dark humid weather, some 500 miles off.

Thursday 27th—Passed Christmas Island at 3 P. M.

Friday 28th—Got up steam at 9 A. M., Java in sight. Rounded Java Head at $4^1/_2$ P. M.; at $2^1/_2$ A. M. anchored off Angier Point.

Saturday 29th—In morning, boats coming off with provisions. Sent ashore at 9 A. M. Up steam, very hot sea, smooth in a very dangerous archipelago. At 6 P. M., anchored near small island. 8 P. M., an immense Banyan, passed Bay of Bantam. At night, by moonlight, had a grand dance.

Sunday 30th—At $10^1/_2$ A. M. , anchored in Batavia Roads. Many ships near. At 4 P. M., in ship's boat and off to city. Went two miles to canal. Up canal a mile, by carriage for five miles to "Hotel des Indes." Found large party at dinner at $6^1/_2$.

OCTOBER—1860

Monday 1st—Up early to Bacte, in garden filled with trees & birds.

Tuesday 2nd—At 4 P. M., left Hotel, came down to landing.

Wednesday 3rd—Japanese had grand breakfast on shore $1700 cost and off to ship.

Thursday 4th—Got under way to "Onrust," small island to coal ship. In evening left, in evening for city. Went to Hotel Marine.

Sunday 7th—At $4^1/_2$, went down to landing, got on the small Goverment Sloop. At $10^1/_2$, got on board.

Monday 8th—Got under way from Onrust, came to old achorage. Many visitors came off. (95 degrees)

Tuesday 9th—many visitors seen off.

Wednesday 10th—At 3 P. M, up anchor for Hong Kong.

Thursday, Friday, Saturday, 18th, 19th and 20th— Heavy seas with the tail wind of a typhoon. Remarkably short and heavy sea.

Sunday 21st—Saw Chinese coast and many junks.

Monday 22nd—At night boarded by Chinese Pilot. At 5 A. M., headed in for Lyee, noon passage. At 9, anchored off Hong Kong. Boarded by an army of Taylors, Souvenirs, curiosity sellers. Got several letters (4), found *Saganaw.*

Tuesday 30th—At 10 A. M. got under way. Steamed out of Harbor.

Wednesday 31st—Fine steaming weather.

NOVEMBER—1860

Thursday 1st—

Tuesday 7th—Westerly, sighted Japan 40 miles off. Blew heavy at night.

Wednesday 8th—At 10 A. M., made Simoda Island—passed the Bay where the Russian frigate was lost by Earthquake. At 2 P. M., made a volcano. At 6, entered Bay of Jeddo. At 9, got ashore having anchored, backed off and anchored for the night.

Friday 9th—Steamed up the Bay, the great peak of Fuji Yama in sight. At 11, stopped off Yokahoma. Sent boat ashore found *Saganaw.* Got under way at 3 P. M. Anchored 7 miles off Jedda. At one time counted 262 Japanese Junks.

Saturday 10th—Embassy left the ship in large junk with all the *accounts.*

Sunday 11th—Pulled 6 miles, landed at Jeddo. Guarded by officials, walked thru the city, came off at night. On board until went ashore 9 A. M.

Friday 16th—Got money changed. Rode to Asakowsa or the Elysian Fields followed by crowds of Japs to Iman Temple. Got back, (met party returning from dinner) to Sioji, had dinner, went into Bazaar.

Saturday 17th—Rode to Hoji—summer garden, got lunch.

Sunday 18th—Rode to Asakowsa, waxworks, theatre, birds & flowers went down to boat. Saw all off, returned to Sioji, dined at Ministers. Rode at night thru Jedda, found all great & deserted at Sioji.

Monday 19th—Up early, had horses ready, after breakfast started for Yokahoma. Rode thru Sinagawa, thru level flat country. Saw numbers of Geese, cranes & ducks. At 4, arrived at Kanagawa, got the boat, went over to Yokahoma, then on board ship.

Tuesday 20th—On board all day.

Wednesday 21st—Ashore purchasing gingers.

Tuesday 27th—Off to Hong Kong, boarded two vessels that evening.

DECEMBER—1860

Wednesday 5th—At 3 P. M., anchored off Hong Kong.

Saturday 8th—On board boat *Williamitter* (*Walcott*) for Canton. Arrived at $5^1/_2$ P. M.

Saturday 15th—Under way for Aden.

Sunday 23rd—At 11 A. M., anchored off Singapore, under way by $10^1/_2$ A. M.

Monday 24th—At 12, met *Dakotah*, stopped got our mail out of her.

Tuesday 25th—CHRISTMAS DAY—In straits of Singapore.

Wednesday 26th—At 7 A. M., we took *Homer*, ships at anchor. Hired her to Penang, paid $100. Left her at $3^1/_2$ P. M.

JANUARY—1861

Tuesday 1st—Beautiful, calm, smooth off Southern part of Ciglas Salli.

Wednesday 2nd—Heavy gale from N. W. all day.

Friday 4th—Passed under steam thru the 90 degree channel in Gulf of Aiden, met school of porpoise one mile long.

Monday 14th—At 2 P. M., anchored off Aiden, a cinder, like Hell-burnt out. At 1 P. M., Fireman killed in town by Black, ship filled with Parsees acting as companions & washermen. Having steamed all the way. Next P. & O. boat leaves on next Saturday for Suez. Went ashore, everything hot, dry & barren. —— Huge, high irregular, dark brown weather-eaten peaks and ranges of mountains lay some three miles off. On

Jack Ass, fine roads. Went thru steamer point past Hotel & two stores and three fire houses on the hills onto a level beach that was well graded near the sea. Up to a keepout in the mountain range, garrisoned by Indian troops and part of regiment of Regular Army. —— mountains to Aiden, found band playing. Started back, went thru very long tunnel thru the base of a high mountain into encampment. The outlet was another deep cut, now dark. Road into Steamer Point. At store bought Dates & Hats. Had next day Miss Thomas & other ladies on board.

Thursday 17th—Rode in dray up to Aiden, saw the Band. Cisterns cut out of solid rock.

Saturday 19th—On shore all day, very hot. Steamed from Mauritius & Calcutta, had arrived, many passengers on shore. In morning, Ward Blanchard, Col. Ripley, & Dr. Macdermit left ship for Suez in steamer. Went aboard steamer. Went onboard steamer ———. Came on board, heavy sea in morning.

Sunday 20th—Mail per Suez, came in. Got letter (M & S) all well, Ship full of *Parsees.*

Monday 21st—Got under way at 6 A. M. Steaming out (coal at $45 per ton) hot in Gulf of Aiden.

Wednesday 23rd—In evening—made high land near Cape Guardafui.

Thursday 24th—This morning, fine wind, N. E. Have smooth, beautiful weather. The high bold precipitous headlands of Cape Guardafui, the W. E. point of Africa in sight all day. The finest headland I ever saw.

FEBRUARY—1861

Sunday 3rd—Passed Comoro Islands, fine wind going 7 Knots. Had heavy rain. Now entering Mozambique channel.

Monday 4th—Dark & rainy. Heavy squall.

Tuesday 5th—Directly under sun, shadows on deck are small and nearly circular, the hottest day I ever felt.

21st—Anchored off Cape Town, heavy fog, on 10th under way, stood in.

MARCH—1861

Saturday 9th—Sailed this evening, Saturday for Boston—steam.

Saturday 30th—Crossed the Equator at 30 degrees today.

APRIL—1861

April 23rd—Anchored at 5, off Boston Light. For the first time got news of the Civil War in the U. S. The capture of Fort Sumpter [*sic*].

April 24th—The new oath offered the officers. Nine of us refused it:
    Engineers Williamson & Ramsay
    Lieutenants Green—U. S. Marine Corps
    E. G. Reed—Midshipman
    D. B. Conrad—Surgeon
    A. N. Brown—Lieutenant
    D. P. McConkie—Lieutenant
were ordered "to leave vessel"
        visited Mrs. B. that evening

25th—Mr. & Mrs. B. & myself on board R. R. train for New York. Detectives arrested me in cars, taken by Order of Governor Andrews for Treason, went under care of Police to Mayor's Office, there got privilege of being put under naval care, being as yet a U. S. officer, not having as yet resigned. Commander Hudson, at navy yard, Boston sent me on board the *Ohio*, receiving ship, under arrest. Was allowed to go to the city on Parole, remained until dismissed by Secretary Welles.

MAY—1861

May 12th—then escaped the Police who kept watch over me, by means of Surgeon Miller and Mr. Batchellor and leaving the city, arrived in New York on 16th.

May 20th—arrived in Harper's Ferry by way of Harrisonburg, Williamsport & Martinsburg. Met by our Picketts at Potomac. Went to Winchester.[4]

Conrad described in his diary his return from Japan with another entry:

Arrived in Boston April 15th, heard of War for the first time. Refused Oath on Board, was ordered 'to leave,' to go anywhere. Tried to do so on 16th, was arrested at Depot. In cars, taken to Mayor who by Governor Anderson's order, sent me to jail for Treason. Got leave to be put under Naval Authority. At navy yard, was put on board *North Carolina* by Commander Hudson. Remained there six weeks, was dismissed by Department for Navy and escaped from yard and got into Virginia by Harrisonburg, Williamsport & Martinsburg...[5]

The log of the *Niagara* on April 25, described this incident at Boston Harbor this way: "The following officers left the ship—Lieut. J. N. Brown, Chief Eng. Wm. P. Williamson, Lieuts. of Marines, I. Green and G. J. Butler, Dr. D. B. Conrad, 1st Asst. Eng. H. A. Ramsey, Mid. E. G. Reed, and Lt. D. P. McCorkle. The first having resigned and the rest declining to take the Oath of Allegiance to the U.S. which the revolutionary attitude of the Southern States had rendered necessary." The log of April 29, stated, "at 6, called all hands to muster, administered the Oath of Allegiance to the U. S." On the April 30, other marines having refused to take the oath were sent under guard to the navy-yard, W. W. Cox, Jno. Miller, J. R. McNeely and R. H. Wiley.[6]

Upon learning of his son's arrest, Robert Young Conrad wrote the following letter to the governor of Virginia:

Winchester, May 4, 1861

To Gov. Letcher—

Dear sir,

My son, Doctor Daniel B. Conrad, a past ass't. Surgeon in the U. S. Navy was arrested in Boston, by order of Gov. Andrews, & is now a prisoner on the *U. S. Receiving Ship Ohio* in Boston Harbor.

He arrived about 10 days ago in Boston in the *U. S. S. Niagara* from Japan & China, and as far as I can learn is now confined, simply on his refusal to take some test oath.

The inclosed letter contains all the information I have and as I wrote to you concerning him when in Richmond. I take the liberty to send this in order to account for you not hearing from him now.

I have written to the Att'y Gen'l of the U. S., Mr. Bates to ask some information on the subject.

I am utterly at a loss to know what is meant by holding him as a hostage for officers confined [in the] South or why the Gov. of Mass. should have arrested him.

Ver. Res'y

Yours

Robert Y. Conrad[7]

Dr. Conrad escaped detention in Boston and arrived on Virginia soil before any intervention was necessary by the governor of Massachusetts.

Chapter Three

Dr. Daniel Burr Conrad, Confederate Naval Surgeon, at the Battle of First Manassas

The state of Virginia established a provisional navy on April 27, 1861, by an ordinance authorizing a force of two thousand officers, seamen and marines.[1] Because of Conrad's experience in the Federal navy, he was appointed a "Passed Surgeon in the Virginia Navy" on May 25, 1861, by Conrad's ex-shipmate, William F. Patton, now surgeon in charge in Richmond. Conrad's appointment read:

> Office of the Bureau of
> Medicine & Surgery
> Richmond May 25th 1861
>
> Sir
> The Governor having appointed you a Passed Assistant Surgeon in the Virginia Navy, I have the pleasure to enclose herewith your Commission bearing date May 23d 1861.
> As you state in your letter to the Governor that you are on duty at Harper's Ferry, you will consider yourself on the same duty until further orders.
>
> Very Respectfully
> Your obt Servant
> Wm F. Patton
> Surgeon in charge
>
> To Passed Ass't Surgeon
> D. B. Conrad
> Virginia Navy
> Winchester, Va.[2]

The Virginia navy existed for only about five weeks, because "by proclamation of the Governor, dated June 6, 1861, 'all officers, seamen, and marines of the Provisional Navy of Virginia,' were transferred to the Confederate States."[3]

Conrad was assigned as surgeon to the 2nd Virginia Volunteer Infantry on June 8, 1861. Conrad told of his first military experiences in a monograph titled "The History of the First Battle of Manassas and the Organization of the Stonewall Brigade; How It Was So Named," published in the *Southern Historical Society Papers*.

When in May, 1861, General Joseph E. Johnston arrived at Harper's Ferry to command the unformed, disorganized mass of men and muskets there assembled, he found five Virginia regiments and two or three from Alabama and Mississippi, all in nominal control, simply by seniority, of a Colonel Jackson of the 'Virginia Army.' Soon order grew out of chaos, and we of the 'Virginia Army' found ourselves one May day on Bolivar Heights, five regiments in all assembled and called the 'Virginia Brigade'; they were the Second, Thirty-third, Twenty-first, Twenty-seventh, and Fourth. Our senior colonel was a man who never spoke unless spoken to; never seemed to sleep; had his headquarters under a tree; the only tent used was that of his adjutant. He walked about alone, the projecting visor of his blue cap concealing his features; a bad-fiting, single-breasted blue coat, and high boots covering the largest feet ever seen, completed his picture. Cadets from the Virginia Military Institute called him 'Old Jack'; told us that he had been of the United States Army in the Mexican war, and had resigned; then was chosen professor of mathematics, and had married a professor's daughter.

He was as exact in the performance of his duties as a mathematical proposition; his only pleasure, walking daily at the same hour for his health; strict, grim and reticent, he imagined that the halves of his body did not work and act in accord. He followed hydropathy for dyspepsia, and after a pack in wet sheets every Sunday morning he then attended the Presbyterian church, leading the choir, and the prayer-meetings every night during the week. He ate the queerest food, and he sucked lemons constantly; but where he got them during the war, for we were many miles from a lemon, no one could find out— but he always had one. In fact, no one knew or understood him. No man ever saw him smile—but one woman, his wife. But he stood very high in the estimation of all for his rigid moral conduct and the absolute faith reposed in his word and deeds. Soon it was observed that every night there was singing and praying under 'that tree,' and every Sunday morning and evening he held prayer-meetings, which, I regret to say, were attended by only a few—always strictly, however, by his staff, who seemed to have been chosen or elected because they were of his way of life. When thrown with him on duty he was uniformly courteous to all. He always kept his eyes half-closed as if thinking, which he invariably did before answering; but his replies were short and to the point. Not many days elapsed before the officers found out that when he gave or wrote one of his short orders, it was always to be obeyed, or suspension at once followed neglect. In May many regiments arrived from Georgia, Mississippi, Alabama and Tennessee, and there was some semblance of discipline— as an immense log guard-house, always filled, gave evidence.

One Sunday evening in early June the long roll was beaten, and we soon were in line, marching out between the high hill towards Shepherdstown bridge on the upper Potomac, accompanied by a long procession of carriages filled with our mothers and sisters, escorted by our middle-aged, portly fathers on horse-back; for as we could not go to them, so they daily visited us in our camp; and that evening, for the first time in our lives, it looked and felt like war. For were we not on our way to keep the Yankees out of Virginia? Were they not in force somewhere in Maryland, intending to cross over the bridge which we were marching to, to defend and burn? This was the feeling and belief of all of us; and as in the narrow country road winding around the many high hills our long line of bright bayonets glinted in the setting sun, our five full regiments, numbering nearly four thousand five hundred of the brightest, healthiest, and the most joyous of Virginia youth, stepping out quickly to the shrill music of the drum and fife, with its accompanying procession of vehicles carrying weeping mothers and sisters, it was my first and most vivid sight of what war might be. As darkness fell apace, all were left behind but the soldiers. It was our first night-march, and by two o'clock we were 'dead beat!' Many fell asleep by the roadside, and were only aroused by the rattling of muskets, as the foremost regiment fired a volley without orders, and swept across the bridge, only to be sternly ordered back by 'Old Jack, the sleepless,' who reprimanded its colonel and then personally superintended the firing of the wooden structure. During the next week we marched over several counties, and by the time we reached Winchester, where General J. E. Johnston had established his headquarters, we were in perfect trim, and knew each other well and felt like soldiers.

In Winchester we were regaled day and night with the speeches of 'Fire-eaters,' 'Original Secessionists,' *Et id genus omne!* I only recall the following: I saw a crowd listening eagerly with arrested attention to an orator. He was both corpulent and crapulent, who had just come from Washington, which was his present glory and distinction. He announced that he would redden the Potomac with the blood of every Yankee who crossed to invade the sacred soil of the South. One Southern man with a bowie knife was equal to any two Yankees, and that the war would be over after the first fight, when they would be driven out and away forever. Another orator drew a large audience; his chief distinction and glory seemed to be that he was and had been a 'Nullifier' (whatever that was). An original 'Secessionist,' had a brother fighting in Italy with Garabaldi, who he announced was expected daily—the looked-for 'Military Messiah,' and finally that he was a South Carolinian and come here to assist in fighting Virginia's battles. Then there were groans and derision from the assembled Virginians.

For a week ending July 2d, we were encamped near Martinsburg, for four miles from the ford of the Potomac leading to Hagerstown, called Falling Waters, watching the Federal army under General [Robert] Patterson. At sunrise the alarm was given: 'the enemy are crossing!' and we were under arms on our way to the ford. Emerging on the turnpike, we were halted to support a battery; skirmishers were thrown out, and soon we were all engaged. We tried hard to hold Patterson until General Johnston could come up from Winchester, but were forced back, and here we saw Colonel Jackson under fire for the first time; stolid, imperturbable, undisturbed, as he was watched by every eye; and his example was quieting and of decided moral effect. There, for the first time, we saw the long line of blue, with the United States flag in the center, and both sides exchanged shots; the first of the many fights in the old Valley of Virginia. We fell back through Martinsburg; it was occupied by General Patterson; and at a small hamlet called 'Bunker Hill,' some seven miles away, we, during the whole of July 4th, were in line of battle, expecting Patterson hourly. The next evening we fell back upon Winchester, and after our arrival there happened an episode which I will relate briefly, as it was the first and only attempt at a mutiny ever heard of in the Confederate army.

About 3 o'clock on the afternoon of July 17th the long roll was beaten and we were marched to an adjoining field, crushing under our feet as we moved along the stone fences bounding it. There we found our five regiments surrounding a number of tents, and when the hollow square was perfect we became aware that we enclosed a battalion of troops who had refused positively to further obey their commander. General Joe Johnston's adjutant, Colonel Whiting, with Colonel Jackson and the colonel of the refractory troops, rode up into the square. The drums were ordered to beat the assembly, and, to our infinite relief, the battalion, under the command of its several captains, fell into line at once. Then there was a dead silence. This was a mutiny! What came next? How was it to be punished? Was every tenth man to be shot, or only the officers? As I rode along I heard these questions asked by both rank and file. Colonel Whiting then rode to the front with a paper in his hand, and when he arrived at the head of the troops he read aloud, with marked emphasis, in substance as follows: That General Johnston had heard with regret and surprise that, on the eve of an action, both men and officers had refused to obey the orders of their commander. He could only say that it was the imperative duty of all soldiers to obey orders; that their grievances would be redressed in time, but such an example would and should not go unpunished. He therefore expected of them instant obedience of their colonel's orders; that Colonel Jackson, with five regiments, was there to enforce, if needed, his commands.

Their own colonel then put them through their evolutions for so many minutes, and they were ordered back to their tents, and all was quiet. It seems hardly necessary to state that those were the last orders ever given by that colonel, as he was removed from command.

All of General Johnston's army were then encamped around Winchester, when, on the 18th of July, at 3 o'clock in the afternoon, again the long roll was sounded. From the number of mounted officers and men galloping furiously off to every encampment, it was evident that there was important news. General Patterson was known to be at Charlestown, twenty miles to the east, but nearer to the passes of the Blue Ridge than we were. General Beauregard was known to be at Manassas station, far to the east, eighty miles by direct line, with the Blue Ridge and the Shenandoah river running between him and us. Soon the news came—it was not an order, but simply a message from General Johnston to each brigade, regiment and individual soldier, that General Beauregard had just notified him from Manassas, on that morning at daybreak, he had been attacked by an overwhelming force of the enemy from Centerville. He was holding his own, but needed help. General Johnston had started, and would go day and night to his relief; and he expected every man who wanted to fight the enemy would up and follow. There is no man living of all that army today who can ever forget the thrill of 'Berseeker rage' which took possession of us all when the news was understood, and General Johnston's inspiring message was repeated along the line. We were to help

General Beauregard drive the enemy back; then, returning to the Valley, would hurl General Patterson across the Potomac and end the war. For had not Secretary Seward proclaimed that in sixty days it would be over.

Every man sprang to his place, and in an incredibly short time we were rapidly moving through the dusty streets of old Winchester, there only to be the more inspired and encouraged, for there was not a mother or sister there who had not in the ranks a son or a brother, and who through tears and wails at being left undefended and alone, yet told us it was our duty to go.

Our Virginia brigade took the lead and to the eastward, making for Ashby's Gap. We footed it fast and furious; it was at first like a run, but soon slackened to the 'route step,' and now we wondered at the old soldier's puzzle: 'Why, when the leading files of a mile of soldiers were only in a walk, that the rear files are always on a run?' As we passed through the rich and fertile Clarke county, the road was lined with ladies holding all manner of food and drink, for General Johnston's staff had passed in a sweeping gallop and given tidings of our coming. At sundown we came to the cold, swift Shenandoah, and with two or three to every horse, the rest stripped off trousers, crossed, holding aloft on muskets and head, clothing and ammunition. This was the severest test, for it was a long struggle against a cold, breast-high current, and the whole night and the next day witnessed this fording of men, guns and horses. I did not see my mare for two days; nearly a dozen cousins and brothers or other relatives had to use her in the crossing. Luckily the road beyond was hard, dry and plain in the dark night as we slowly climbed the Blue Ridge, which rises precipitously from the river, and in a straggling line passed by the 'Big Poplar Tree' that crowns the summit and is the corner of four counties, Clark, Warren, Fauquier and Loudoun.

Coming down the mountain by the hamlet of Paris, and there leaving the pike, we took the country road, soft and damp, to the railroad station of Piedmont, where, sleeping on the ground, we awaited the arrival of the train to carry us to Manassas Junction. At sunrise it came; a long train of freight and cattle cars, in which we packed ourselves like so many pins and needles; and, as safety for engine and cars was more essential than speed, for we had one engine only on that part of the old Manassas Gap Railroad, we slowly jolted the entire day, passed the many

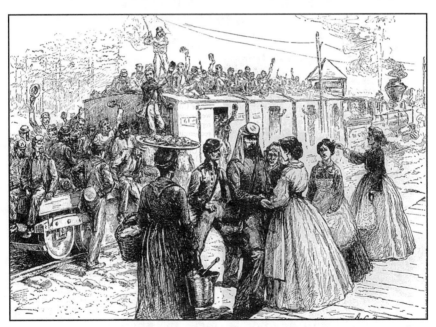

2nd Virginia Regiment Arrives at Manassas

Depicts the ladies of Manassas greeting the regiment with refreshments, the nine thousand Confederates under General Joseph E. Johnston. Dr. Conrad was among these men arriving for the impending Battle of First Manassas.

Battles and Leaders

country stations, warmly welcomed by the gathered crowds of women and girls with food and drink.

And when at sunset we arrived at Manassas Junction, sprung at once into lie, and swept out into a broken country of pine forest. Four miles brought us to the banks of 'Bull Run,' where we slept. That was Friday night, the 19th, and it had taken twenty-four hours to bring four thousand men to the expected field of action.

Bright and early on Saturday, the 20th, we were up and examined with a soldier's interest the scene of the conflict of the 18th. A line of fresh graves was rather depressing; the trees were lopped and mangled by shot and perforated by minnie balls. The short, dry grass showing in very many spots a dark chocolate hue, spreading irregularly like a map, which the next day became a too familiar sight. We could not make anything out of the fight, beyond that here was the ford, and here they came down to cross in force. They were simply repulsed from the ford; there was no pursuit, the artillery remaining on the hills beyond; and it was agreed that here, any day now, we were to fight against a direct assault. The enemy's object, we supposed, was to get to Manassas Junction, murder every one there, and destroy buildings and stores. The art of war was so simple and so well understood by all in those early days, that the opinions of high-up college graduates and successful lawyers were even sought for, and in all cases, I must do them justice to say, were given with the utmost freedom and liberality. Every man who had been in the Mexican War, or had been fighting abroad, was a colonel or a brigadier at once, and they swelled and swaggered around, dispensing willing information of tactics and grand strategy in the most profuse and generous way to an absorbent and listening crowd.

The whole of Saturday, the 20th, did we lie in the pines, resting and surmising, greeting each new regiment as it arrived at all hours of the day and night, panting for the fight. Questions asked were: 'Had the fighting begun yet?' 'Are we too late?' 'When was it to be? Let us get a good place where we can kill every d—— d Yankee, and then go home.' Not a sound or shot distured the quiet of long Saturday, and we slept peacefully in the pines that night. As the next day (Sunday, the 21st) broke we were jumped out of our lairs by the loudest gun I ever heard, apparently fired right at our heads, as we supposed, and from just over the bank of Bull Run, only a hundred yards distant; but it proved to be the signal gun from Centerville, four miles away, in the encampment of General McDowell. At a double quick we were in line along the bank of the stream, momentarily expecting the enemy to appear and open on us, and thus we awaited until the sun got over the tops of the trees, when a mounted officer rode up, and after a hurried interview with Colonel Jackson, we were, to our surprise, wheeled to the rear, and at double-quick, over fields and through the woods, we went to the extreme left of our army. It then turned out that at that day and hour General McDowell had decided to attack us on our left; and as General Beauregard had decided to attack the Federals on their left, so, had it not been discovered in time by the Confederates, each army would have followed thereto in concentric circles. For two long, hot hours did we move to wards the rattling of musketry, which at first was very faint, then became more and more audible. At last we halted under a long ridge covered with small pines. Here were the wounded of that corps who had been first engaged—men limping on gun or stick; men carried off in blankets, bleeding

their life away; men supported on each side by soldiers—and they gave us no very encouraging news
to troops as we were. They had been at it ever since
sun-up. The enemy were as thick as wheat in the field,
and the long lines of blue could not be counted. Up
the narrow lane our brigade started, directly to where
the musketry seemed the loudest, our regiment, the
Second, bringing up the rear. Reaching the top, a wide
clearing was discovered; a broad table land spread
out, the pine thicket ceased, and far away over the
hill in front was the smoke of musketry; at the bottom of the long declivity was the famous turnpike,
and on the hills beyond could be seen clearly Griffin's
and Rickett's batteries. In their front, to their rear,
and supported on each side, were long lines of blue.
To our right, about one hundred yards off, was a
small building, the celebrated 'Henry House.' As ours
was the last regiment to come up, and as the brigade, as it surmounted the hill, wheeled into line
sharply to the left into the thickets, we were thus
thrown to the extreme right of the line and of the
entire army. Halting there and mounted on a gate-
post, I could see the panoramas spread out before
me. The brass pieces of Griffin's and Rickett's batteries were seen wheeling into line, caissons to the
rear, the horses detached and disappearing behind
the hill. The glinting of the morning sun on the bur-
nished metal made them very conspicuous. No cavalry were seen. I do not think that McDowell had any
in action that day. Both batteries soon opened on us
with shell, but no casualties resulted, for the reason
that in their haste and want of time the fuses were
not cut. I picked up many which fell to the ground
with a dull sound, and found that the reason they
did not explode.

The infantry were engaged on the side of the long,
gradual slope of the hill on which we stood, and in

the bottom below, out of our sight, we could hear the sound and see the white smoke. At this time there rode up fast towards us from the front a horse and rider, gradually rising to our view from the bottom of the hill. He was an officer all alone, and as he came closer, erect and full of fire, his jet-black eyes and long hair, and his blue uniform of a general officer made him the cynosure of all. In a strong, decided tone he inquired of the nearest aide, what troops we were and who commmanded. He was told that Colonel Jackson, with five Virginia regiments had just arrived, and pointed to where the colonel stood at the same time. The strange officer then advanced, and we of the regimental staff crowded to where he was to hear the news from the front. He announced himself as General B. E. Bee, commanding South Carolina troops; he said that he had been heavily engaged all the morning, and being overpowered, are now slowly being pushed back; we will fall back on you as a support; the enemy will make their appearance in a short time over the crest of that hill. 'Then sir, we will give them the bayonet,' was the only reply of Colonel Jackson. With a salute, General Bee wheeled his horse and disappeared down the hill, where he immortalized himself, Colonel Jackson and his troops, by his memorable words to his own command: 'Close up, men, and stand your ground. Colonel Jackson with five regiments of Virginia troops is standing behind us like a stonewall, and will support you.'

Thus was the name of 'Stonewall' given to General Jackson and his famous brigade. General Bee was killed the next moment.

Our entire line lay in the pine thickets for one long hour, and no man, unless he was there, can tell how very long it was to us. Under fire from two batteries throwing time-shells only, they did not do a great amount of killing, but it was terribly demoralizing. Then there was a welcome cessation; and we were wondering why, and when the fighting would begin for us. After nearly half an hour the roar of the field pieces sounded louder than I had yet heard, and evidently very near us; this was the much criticized movement of Rickett's, who had ordered his battery down the opposite hill, across the pike and up the hill we were on, where, wheeling into battery on the level top, opened with grape and canister right into the thicket and into our exposed line. This was more than Colonel Jackson could stand, and the general order was—'Charge and take that battery!' Now the fight of Manassas, or Bull Run, began in earnest—for the position we held was the key of the field. Three times did our regiment charge up to and take this battery, but never held it; for though we drove the regiment supporting it, yet another was always close behind to take its place. A grey-headed man, sitting sideways on horseback, whom I understood to be General Heintzleman, was ever in one spot directing the movements of each regiment as it came up the hill; and his coolness and gallantry won our admiration. Many fragments of these regiments charged on us in turn as we retreated into the pines, only to be killed, for I do not think any of them went back alive. The green pines were filled with the Seventy-ninth Highlanders and the red-breeched Brooklyn Zouaves, but the only men who were killed twenty or thirty yards behind, and in the rear of our line, were the United States Marines. Many of these I had sailed with, and they called on me by name to help them as they lay wounded in the undergrowth. 'Water, water!' 'Turn me over!' 'Raise my head, and remove me out of this fire!' were their cries. I then saw what was afterwards too often the case—men with wounded legs, unable to move out of the fire, mortally wounded while lying helpless.

Our entire brigade thus fought unaided and alone for at least an hour—charging, capturing, retreating, and retaking this battery, resisting the charges of each fresh regiment as it came forward at quick-step up the slope of the hill, across the table-land, on its top and into the pine thickets where we were, until we were as completely broken up into fragments and as hard pressed as men ever were. It had gotten down to mere hand-to-hand fighting of small squads, out in the open and in the pines. There was no relief, no reinforcements, no fresh troops to come, or to fall back on. Luckily the enemy were in the same disorganized condition as we were. General Johnston seized the colors of a regiment, and on horseback, let a charge, excusing it afterwards as necessary at that moment to make a personal example. Our Colonel Jackson, with only two aides, Colonels Jones and Marshall, both subsequently killed, rode slowly, and without the slightest hurrah, frequently along our front, encouraging us by his quiet presence. He held aloft his left or bridle hand, looking as if he was invoking a blessing, as many supposed, but in fact to ease the intense pain, for a bullet had badly shattered two of his fingers, to which he never alluded, and it has been forgotten, for it was the only time he was ever wounded, until his fall in action in 1863.

Thus the fate of the field hung in a balance at 2:30 P. M. At this moment President Davis and his staff made their appearance on the field, but not being known, attracted no attention. Both sides were exhausted and willing to say 'enough!' The critical moment, which comes in all actions, had arrived, when we saw to our left a cloud of dust. As they passed by and through our squads there were hurried inquiries; the enemy was pointed out to them, and when seen, from out of their dusty and parched throats, came the first 'Rebel yell.' It was a fierce, wild cry, perfectly involuntary, caused by the emotion of catching first sight of the enemy. These new troops were Kirby Smith's delayed men; the train had that morning broken down, but on arriving at the station near and hearing the sound of fighting, he had ordered the strain stopped, and forming into line and rapidly marching, guided only by the roar of the guns, had arrived on the field at the supreme moment.

The 'yell' attracted the attention of the enemy, surprised and startled them. Inspired by the sight of the Federals the new Confederate troops, in one long line, with a volley and another yell, swept down the slope of our hill and drove before them the broken, tired enemy, who had been at it since sunrise. Kirby Smith was shot from his horse, but onward they went, irresistible, for there was no opposition. The enemy stood for a few moments, firing, then turned their backs for the first time. As if by magic the whole appearance of the scene was changed. One side was cheering and pursuing in broken, irregular lines; the other a slow-moving mass of 'blue backs' and legs, guns, caissons and ammunition wagons, started down the hard, white pike. Our batteries, with renewed vigor and dash, had again come to the front, and from their high positions were opening with shot and grape.

One solitary bridge was the point to which the fleeing Federals converged, and on that point was our fire concentrated. The result was at once seen— a wheel or two knocked off their caissons or wagons blocked the passage, and the bridge became impassable. The men cut loose their horses, mounted and rode away; others plunged into the mud and water, and the retreat became from that moment a panic, for the god Pan had struck them hard for the first and last time. There was never again the like to be seen in the subsequent four years.

Our pursuit, singularly, was by artillery, our infantry having become incapable of further motion from sheer exhaustion; and Stewart had only a few companies out of the one regiment on the field; but they did good work in keeping up the rout until late in the night, when they were brought to a standstill at Centerville, where there was a reserve brigade that had not been in action; and so ended the part taken by the Stonewall Brigade in this their first fight. I may add here that our regiment was not gathered together for four days, and the brigade not for a week. With us, as with the rest of our victorious army, we were as much disorganized and scattered by our victory as the Federals by their defeat, and pursuit, unless by an organized force beyond Centerville, would have been simply a physical impossibility.[4]

Conrad took part in the search for the body of Colonel Francis J. Thomas, killed at First Manassas. Thomas had taken over the command of the regiment of infantry known as Wheat's Tigers after Major Chatham Roberdeau Wheat had been wounded early in the battle. This episode was related in the memoirs of Dr. E. A. Craighill.

The day the battle of Manassas was fought the sun was scorching hot, but a short time after dark it commenced raining quite briskly, a condition which I often noticed later, following heavy cannonading. It was between 10 and 11 after I was through, as I thought, for the night with dead and wounded comrades, when I was told that my cousin, Colonel Francis J. Thomas, said to have been promoted that day as Brigadier General had been killed commanding 'Wheat's Tigers,' Major Wheat, their commander, having been badly wounded early in action. The Tigers were a desperate set of 'Warf rats' from New Orleans. Col. Thomas was Johnston's chief of ordnance, a classmate of Jackson at West Point and I think a close friend...was desperately wounded and left on the field for dead...When Wheat was wounded his 'Tigers,' tough as they were, became very much demoralized and General Johnston requested Colonel Thomas to take command of them and lead them in their charge. (An ordnance officer as a rule does not command fighting soldiers.) While leading this charge I was told he was killed, but I did not know of it until the battle was over late at night. To find his body I started out with a lantern. I had seen 'cousin Frank' that morning, a picture of health and not forty years old. I got general directions from a surgeon in our command whom I knew, Dr. Dan Conrad, an old Navy surgeon, so I started with my lantern. It was very dark, and it seemed to me I must have stumbled over a hundred dead men before I reached the point Dr. C. had indicated, but did not find Colonel Thomas' body. It must have been removed, or I did not find the place. I then walked over the field hoping to find him, and do not know how many dead I turned over, hoping by the light of the lantern to recognize his dead face. I was not successful, and after what seemed hours of this gruesome experience, I gave it up as hopeless, and returned to the Pringle house tired, sleepy, hungry, hoping to get a mouthful of food and a place to sleep,—I was not particular about either. I renewed my search the next day with the aid of daylight to help me. I faithfully walked all over the field and never succeeded in finding the object of my search, and to this day, so far as I know, no one has ever been able to say where he was buried, or if he was buried at all, although I heard afterwards why my search on the night of the battle and the following day had been so unsuccessful.

It seemed that Dr. Conrad, who knew Colonel Thomas well, had seen his body just as he told me, 'lying on his back dressed in blue uniform (likely the one he wore in Mexico) with no indication of his rank, but on the breast of his coat was a paper pinned giving his name and rank, and over his body muskets were stacked, showing he was an officer of high rank.' Dr. C. was thus minute in giving me directions. After long weeks when I saw Dr. Conrad again he explained that when the burying detail was sent out after the battle to get together and bury the dead, the instructions were to carry the body of Colonel Thomas to Johnston's headquarters to be buried the next day, but by some mistake the men carried it to Beauregard's headquarters; and as there was nothing on him to designate his rank, the pinned on paper being misplaced or lost, his body was carried out and buried without having been recognized, though he was well known to both Johnston and Beauregard, neither of whom very likely ever thought of Colonel Thomas. After a battle is awful![5]

After the battle, but while still at Manassas, Dr. Conrad filed the following requisition:

Special Requisition

Med. Director:

Sir

There is required for the use of the Medical Department of the 2nd Reg't Va. Vols.

One Ambulance

Two mules or horses

Two sets of harnesses

I certify the above requisition...the articles specified are absolutely requisite for the public service rendered to us by the following circumstance.

D. B. Conrad

Surgeon, C. S. Navy

Approved: Thos. H. Williams
              Surgeon, C.S.A.
              Medical Director
              Army Potomac

Received at Manassas Junction from Lt. C. McRae Selph, A.A.Q.M., C.S.A. on the 15th day of August 1861.

(1) one ambulance
(2) Two Horses
(2) " Sets Harnesses

A. S. Stonebraker
Q. M. 2nd Regt Va. Inf.[6]

At First Manassas, Daniel Conrad lost two cousins who were the sons of David Holmes Conrad. Holmes Addison Conrad and Henry Tucker Conrad were killed by the same Federal volley on July 21. Henry Tucker had been a student at the University of Virginia and Holmes Addison had been a student at Episcopal Theological Seminary. They both enlisted on the first of May, in Company D of the 2nd Virginia Regiment of Stonewall's Brigade. They were both buried in the Old Norborne Cemetery in Martinsburg, in what is now West Virginia.

Surgeon Conrad was camped near Bull Run at Centreville, when he was ordered to become the president of the Medical Examining Board which evaluated the qualifications of would-be Confederate army doctors.

On August 13, 1861, Dr. Conrad asked to be detached from the 2nd Virginia Regiment Volunteers:

Headquarters

Gen. Jos. Johnston
    Commander Army of Potomac
        Sir

I respecfully request to be detached from the 2nd Reg't Va. Vols. of which I

am at present acting Surgeon and apply for orders
to hospital at Manassas Springs or the University of
Va.

Respectfully
Your Obt Servant
D. B. Conrad

August 13th 1861   Surgeon, C.S. Navy[7]

Two weeks later, Dr. Conrad was ordered to report to the
medical director's office at Manassas Junction following the
arrival of his replacement:

Medical Director's Office
Manassas Junction, Va.
August 31st, 1861

Special Orders
   No. 23.
          Surgeon J. P. Smith P.A.C.S. is assigned to
duty as Surgeon of the 2nd Reg't Va. Vols.
   He will proceed without delay to Camp Harmon,
near Centreville and report to the Colonel of the
Regiment for duty.
   Upon the arrival of Surgeon Smith, Surgeon D. B.
Conrad, C.S.N. will report to the office for duty.

Thos. H. Williams
Surgeon C.S.A.

Medical Director Army of Potomac

For:
   Surg'n D. B. Conrad, C.S.N.
      Camp Harmon,
         Va.[8]

Surgeon James P. Smith would, later in the war, hold the
lamp while surgery was performed on General Jackson by Dr.
Hunter McGuire at the Wilderness.[9]

   Dr. Conrad received the following letter from one of his
friends, Mary Morris Marshall, who offered to help him in
his treatment of the wounded that survived the battle at
Manassas:

                                          Mount Blanc
                                      September 19th

Dr. Conrad
    Dear Sir
        I take the liberty of sending you a few lines,
begging you will let me know if I can be in any way
of assistance to you in your attendance upon the sick.
I have sent various articles by different ways to the
sick, but know of only one case in which the pack-
age reached the persons intended for. Are you in need
of ice? We hear contradictory reports such as that
ice is much needed & then that the boxes of ice sent
down in the soldiers' car will return up the road untouched. My mind has been much exercised upon
the subject of the sick at Manassas & I was so very
glad to day to hear that you will [be] of the Drs. attending there. In as I felt sure I might apply to you
with hope of receiving reliable information as to what
was needed and where to send it. I shall give this to
my Mother to inclose in a note she intends writing
you. I hope if your duties, gives you any respite, you
will come for a rest to pay us a visit. You might not
be able to spare time to go to your own home. When
you could take a day or so to come to Markham Station where we would meet you. I shall always be glad
to see you at Mount Blanc as well as to render you
any assistance in any province.
                        Your sincere friend
                        M. M. Marshall

On the back of this letter is written:

    Letter from Mary Morris Marshall of 'Mt. Blanc,'
Markam, Va., to my father Dr. D. B. Conrad; just after the first battle of Manassas, in the Civil War. [The
above] Written by Annie Conrad Little.[10]

In September, Conrad was ordered by Captain Franklin
Buchanan to Charleston by the Navy Department for duty on

the CSS *Nashville*. Conrad was to report to Flag Officer Duncan Ingraham who had been sent to Charleston to strengthen the naval defenses there.

> Confederate States,
> Office of Orders and Detail,
> Navy Department,
> Richmond, Va. Sept 23rd 1861
>
> Sir:
>
> You are hereby detached from the C. S. Army and you will proceed to Charleston, S. C. forthwith and report to Capt. D. N. Ingraham, for duty.
>
> I am, respectfully,
> Your obedient servant,
> Franklin Buchanan
> Captain in charge.
>
> By command of the Secretary of the Navy.
>
> Surgeon
> Daniel B. Conrad
> C. S. Navy
> Manassas, Virginia
>
> All officers will promptly acknowledge the receipt of orders, and inform the Department immediately on their having reported in obedience to them.[11]

About the time of his receipt of his new orders, Conrad was given the following partially printed pass on September 26, 1861, so that he could proceed from Manassas Junction on official business:

> **QUARTERMASTER'S DEPARTMENT, C.S.A.**
> Manassas Junction, Va., *Sept. 26,* 1861.
> To the Superintendent of the *Manassas Gap* Railroad
> Be pleased to furnish transportation for_*Surgeon*_
> _____*Daniel B. Conrad*_____
> On your railroad from *Manassas to Piedmont and return* on official business.
> *F. N.[?] Powell*, Transportation Agent,
> *Q. M.*[12]

USS *Nashville*

The *Nashville* was a side-wheel, brig-rigged, passenger steamer of 1,221 tonnage. She was 215 feet long with a 35-foot beam. She plied the waters running between New York and Charleston, South Carolina. "After the fall of Fort Sumter she was seized and refitted by the Confederate government. Under the command of Lieutenant Robert B. Pegram, CSN, she braved the blockade on October 21, 1861, and headed out across the Atlantic. On November 19 she captured and burned the American clipper ship *Harvey Birch*, and two days later arrived at Southampton, England, where she was the first ship to fly the Confederate flag in English waters. While the *Nashville* was in dry dock at Southampton, a warship of the US Navy, the USS *Tuscarora*, arrived hoping to engage the rebel cruiser as she put out to sea. British authorities, however, enforced the international law which stated "that 24 hours should elapse before the departure of one belligerent ship in pursuit of another." On February 3, 1862, the *Nashville* escaped and headed for Bermuda and from there to Beaufort, North Carolina, where she again ran the blockade on February 28.

About this time Federal forces under General Ambrose Burnside were moving on Confederate strongpoints in the area, and the *Nashville* was again forced to run the blockade to escape capture. With seeming impunity she ran into Georgetown, South Carolina. The resultant publicity given to the *Nashville* and her ability to elude the Yankee blockade almost at will angered Northerners who called for the resignation of Secretary Gideon Welles. While at Georgetown the *Nashville* was sold to a private concern for use as a blockade runner and renamed the *Thomas L. Wragg*.

On April 24, 1862, she made a successful run into Wilmington, North Carolina, with a cargo of 60,000 stand of arms and 40,000 tons of powder. She did not, oddly enough, remain a blockade runner for long, for on November 5, 1862, she was commissioned as a privateer, armed with two 12-pounders, and renamed *Rattlesnake...*

The *Nashville*, or *Rattlesnake*, was unable to make good her escape and was eventually shut up tight in Ossabaw Sound, Georgia, sheltered beneath the protective guns of Fort McAllister. On February 27, 1863, during a shelling attack on the fort by the USS *Montauk*, Commander John Worden, USN, it was noticed that the big privateer was hard aground. At daylight the following day the Federals returned and, under heavy fire from the fort, began to shell the *Nashville*. Within 20 minutes the ship was in flames, and at 9:30 A.M. blew up." Thus she was lost in the Ogeechee River, near Fort McAllister, Georgia, on February 28, 1863.[13]

In Richmond, Dr. Conrad found that the ironclad *Nashville* had already left the port of Charleston. Dr. Conrad was very lucky he missed the *Nashville* because it would soon be sunk with great loss of life.

Conrad was then ordered to New Orleans by the following order:

> Confederate States
> Office of Orders and Details
> Navy Department
> Richmond Sept. 30th, 1861
>
> Sir
>
> Your order of the 23rd inst. to proceed to Charleston and report to Capt. D. N. Ingraham is hereby revoked and you will proceed to New Orleans and report to Flag Officer G. N. Hollins for duty.
>
> Respectfully
> Your Obt servant
> Franklin Buchanan
> Officer in charge
> by order of Sec. of Navy[14]

Dr. Conrad reported to Hollins in New Orleans on October 14, 1861. The next day, Surgeon Conrad received his $118.80 traveling allowance from Richmond to New Orleans calculated at 10¢ a mile for the 1,188 miles. Here in New Orleans, Daniel saw his brother, Powell, healthy for the last time. He would later see Powell in Richmond when Powell was in his final stages of typhoid fever. Dr. Conrad was told to report to the CSS *Ivy* at the naval rendezvous at New Orleans. Dr. Conrad while in New Orleans wrote the following letter to his brother.

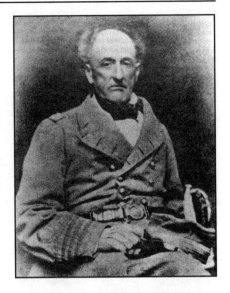

Captain Franklin Buchanan, CSN

As captain in charge of the Office of Orders and Detail Buchanan issued commands by the secretary of the navy.
Charles Lee Lewis,
Admiral Franklin Buchanan

Naval Rendezvous
New Orleans

My Dear Holmes,

From the papers, I imagine you are between F.C.H. [Fairfax Court House] and Centreville and that in your sudden move for lost baggage and tents, also, that we drove the 'Yankee Gangs' back from Leesburg with some loss. I should like to hear the particulars of you. I am on duty here shipping men and surgeons on the receiving ships and fully occupied by day— nothing to do at night. Cannot get into the habit of visiting. Met Charles Conrad one night. Was on sick leave from camp near mouth of Mississippi; belongs to artillery; thinks he was badly sick; wants to get off. What about the advances up the valley. It gave me great uneasiness at the time. Great preparations are being made here for an expected attack on the city. Everybody drilling and afterwards 'drinking and blowing.' Gunboats are being built here also floating batteries. A fleet of iron clad boats are being built in Cincinnati which give some uneasiness and may do mischief to plantations. Already has there been one serious insurrection near Vicksburg. The Negroes awaiting the arrival of Lincoln boats to free them. This is the great trouble here. There exists no more worthless, trifling, emasculated set of men in the wide world than the young cotton and sugar planters of the South. No education, no profession, enervated by dissatisfaction and sloth, lazy, either to act or think. They while away an existence worthy of an Indian or Mexican. Amongst the females only are found all the virtues but no education. You must be growing tired of cavalry. Do you want a change? To what I see nothing better but, can readily get you a berth on board some small steamer if you wish it and by this means you can be free again to choose. It is possible next summer if all is well. I may get up to Va. in the army if possible and so soon as the war is over will apply for a permanent transfer to Army. Do you like Colonel Jones. How does Swann and he get on. It is suppposed here that the seat of war will be transferred to Ky and Missouri. Certainly the hardest fighting will be done there. The finest men in the world are there, on both sides. The west is impatient at having its river blocked up. They are bound by trade and interest to the South but will not join with us. It is surmised they will form ultimately a separate Confederacy.

Saturday:

Just heard of the Leesburg affair. Do write me of any of our relatives here in it. It seems very probable that an advance will be made by [X.] Army down the valley tho I've no good reason why. An iron cased ship driven by two propellers accompanied by three steamers went into the enemy fleet the other night. It is highly probable, almost certain, that the '*Preble*' was sunk, at least so seriously injured, that she will not available for some months. The fleet went up the river to where the Delta begins called the 'Head of the Passes.' They were driven out side and there got. More damage would have been done had not the engine of the so called 'Manassas' been disjointed by the sudden shock. She was going near 10 miles an hour. Drove her nose near 9 feet into something wooden covered with copper, if one may judge by the particles adhering. She is now repairing having a new nose attached. The old one being so slewed as to be unavailable for blows. It is possible you may hear of me next at Columbus on the River or Ky. When the great army is and where the gunboats will be attacked coming down from Cincinnati. A fine one is going up from here, commanded by a friend. Loyall, I see had been arrested and imprisoned in Fort Lafayette for refusing the oath.

Let me hear something of the 2nd Regt. What has become of Clarke and his company. Has Red McGuire gotten an exchange. How is Hunter now. Remember me to Eleason Randolph. Powers and the member of your mess.

Believe me ever yours truly,
D. B. Conrad

Monday
Your letter is past due. Conrad[15]

It is not known when Conrad arrived on board the *Ivy* but the following describes the action in which the *Ivy* participated near that time.

On October 9, the *Ivy* attacked Federal blockaders at the Head of Passes on the Mississippi River. Though unable to inflict major damage on the enemy, her long-range guns caused serious concern among Federal naval commanders. Three days later she again sallied out, accompanied by the ram *Manassas* and the steamer *James L. Day*. The engagement resulted in the grounding of two Yankeee ships as the *Ivy* demonstrated the value of her long-range guns and maneuverability. She remained active in the lower Mississippi until forced back by the weight of Federal naval forces under Admiral Farragut.[16] 'The *Preble* returned to the United States in September 1860, and ten months later joined the Gulf Blockading Squadron. On October 12, 1861, she participated in an engagement with a Confederate naval force led by the *CSS Manassas* near Head of Passes, Mississippi River...[The *Preble*] was accidentally destroyed by fire on April 27, 1863, at Pensacola, Florida.[17]

The following is an interesting letter from Dr. Conrad's father to another son, Holmes, describing the situation down

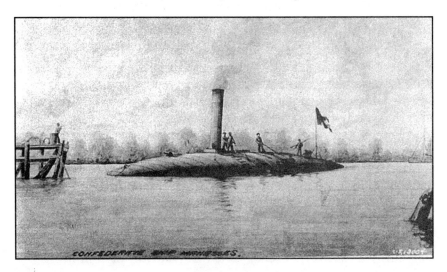

CSS *Manassas*

This very low silhouetted ironclad steamer ram had a 32-pound carronade located in the bow and was protected by armor only an inch and a half thick.

Civil War Naval Chronology, 1861-1865

river from Richmond and stating that Dan is now at New Orleans.

Richmond
30 Nov. 1861

Dear Holmes,

My correspondence on matters of business and with my family (scattered as it is at home, New Orleans, and Manassas), has been so great since our meeting here, that I really could not find time to write to you, although always intending to do so. Our session is, I trust, about to come to a close. We have adopted a new militia system intended to virtually to compel our present volunteer force to renew their enlistments at least for one year; and I think its provisions will have the desired effects. The amendments to the constitution are nearly through with, and although we have failed to carry several important reforms yet great improvements have been made in changing the tenure of judges, lengthening the terms of justices to 12 years, abolishing elections by people of the sheriffs, clerks, constables, etc., and some other respects. By Tuesday or Wednesday next, I hope to be on my way home.

When I first came down, I took a trip of four days down the James River, and upon the Peninsula visiting nearly all the camps and especially Jamestown, Williamsburg and Yorktown. The march of a hostile force overland or even approach by the rivers is, I should think, effectively blocked in that direction; though General McGruder, (who is exceedingly apprehensive of danger to his command), has just sent up for reinforcements and information of a landing by his enemy in Mathews County (between York and Rappahannock Rivers). His fear seems that they intend to march on Richmond and therefore it is necessary for him to break up his camp and follow them.

With deference to his great military judgement, I think they only intend to plunder and annoy, and have made no preparations for a march into the interior.

The Congress now sitting here now is a very intelligent and respectable body, and I have been quite interested in the conversations with Southern members about affairs in their several regions. Charles Conrad and [illegible] are both in town, but owing to the crowd in the city, and our different occupations, I have only seen the former for a few minutes and the last not at all. I more regret my failure to meet with Captain M. F. Maury, with whom I had a good deal of talk when here before. He has called twice to see me during this trip, and I went to his house one evening, but we have not met.

All the recent movements of the enemy whilst they seem almost to tie us hand and foot and have had the effect at lengthening some faces here, really I think, amount to nothing, but proof that they are unable or unwilling to meet our armies in the field in fair fight. Our thousand miles of coast and hundred ports of entry cannot of course be defended against incursions by water. But these give no permanent advantage to the invader, and are probably intended only to furnish material for dressing up in the press and news page. It will be hard to meet Congress next Monday, with the government in all its branches, backed by the grand army blockaded and besieged in their capitol, and the general not daring to move out and attack the besieging force. It seems to me that very soon they will have no alternative but to attack our army or evacuate Washington. The single stem of railroad to Baltimore is the only channel left open to them for supplies. It is wholly insufficient and we hear that already their troops are on short allowance and their horses dying for want of forage. Winter quarters there must be out of the question, unless they can first open the Potomac.

Dan is at New Orleans in charge as Surgeon at the Rendezvous and Receiving Ship. He writes that he is not well and is anxious to get back to the army at Centreville.

Holmes is yet in a cavalry company near Centreville, engaged in daily fights occuring with scouts and skirmishers. The other day one of his men was shot down by his side. He says that he has not faltered in his purpose to continue to the last, but that a large proportion of the volunteers, unless allowed to visit their homes will refuse to serve after their present terms expire. I would ask you to write, but home to be at home before I could hear from You. With love to all of you,

Yours truly,
R. Y. Conrad[18]

On April 29, 1862, Daniel Conrad now in Vicksburg, Mississippi, was ordered to "proceed to Richmond and report to the Hon. Sec. of the Navy for Duty." Conrad arrived in Richmond on May 10, 1862, and received his traveling allowance of $157.60 for the 1,576 miles. He stayed with his brother, Powell, until Powell's death from typhoid fever contracted in camp. Conrad then returned to the 2nd Virginia Regiment and was with Jackson chasing General Banks down the Shenandoah Valley in the retreat up to Cross Keys and Port Republic.

Dr. Hunter McGuire established the precedent early in the war of immediately freeing all captured medical personnel. Dr. Conrad assisted him in this humanitarian gesture as related here by Dr. McGuire:

In the month of May, 1862, after the defeat of General Banks by General Jackson at Winchester, I found among the captured prisoners eight surgeons or assistant surgeons at the Union Hotel Hospital in

Winchester. As Medical Director of the Army I reported the fact to General Jackson and asked his permission to unconditionally release these medical officers upon their parole of honor. They were to remain in charge of the Federal sick and wounded in Winchester for fifteen days. After the expiration of the fifteen days their parole permitted them to report to their commanding officers for duty. It was understood by these gentlemen that they were to use every effort to have released, on the same terms, the medical officers of the Confederate States, who were then prisoners of the Federal Government, or any medical officers of the Confederate States who might thereafter be captured. General T. J. Jackson assented to the proposition I made to him very readily and directed me to carry out the suggestion. With Dr. Daniel B. Conrad of the Second Virginia Regiment, Confederate States, I went to the Union Hotel Hospital and released on parole the surgeons, assistant surgeons, attendants and nurses, but not the sick and wounded who were afterwards paroled by the regular officers of our army, not to take up arms again until properly exchanged...[19]

Below is a letter to Dan from his brother Holmes telling about the conditions at Winchester and the presence of sham fortifications built by the occupying troops.

Dr. Dan,   May 7th
    I made a trip to Win [chester]. Flanked the pickets—surprised them all and returned safely.
    I found all very well. Father looking rather thin but hearing from us all and from the Army did him good.
    The Yanks are behaving very well—not searching or even stealing. They have put up fortifications upon the hill back of Mr. Alf Powell's place which tho having the appearance of being extensive are by

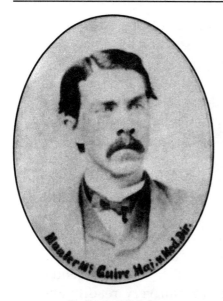

Dr. Hunter McGuire

Dr. McGuire asked his friend, Daniel Conrad, to come and serve with him on Lieutenant General "Stonewall" Jackson's medical staff. McGuire was instrumental in formulating the agreement by both sides of not holding physicians as prisoners of war.

From composite photograph
"Lt. Gen. T. J. Jackson and staff"

a telescope but a sham and put up to terrify the citizens. They muster to kill the time if Jackson entered it. See if our Hughes has gone except Stephen James, and a girl. The people look daily to be delivered by Jackson. They have 300 Yankees and think it terrible to be kept thus by them. Charles is at Staunton. James the provost has promised to let him out on a parole for six months. I advised that he should go to Hartman Bridge. M was wondering what has become of you and the Army.

Your B.

Holmes Conrad[20]

Dr. Conrad was with the Stonewall Brigade when it marched down to Richmond. He was there during the Seven Days' fight, in charge of the Brock House Hospital. He was ordered to Charleston, Savannah, and Mobile on the Examining Board. In Mobile, on September 5, 1862, Conrad was ordered, to "proceed to Richmond and report for duty, to Flag Officer G. N. Hollins, President of Naval Examining Board."

Dr. Conrad's father wrote the following letter to Dan telling of the personal troubles he was having with the occupying forces in Winchester. His father mentioned that he had been arrested and held hostage by the Federal troops. Robert Young Conrad, being one of the more prominent citizens of Winchester, would be arrested a total of three times. He was sent, on one of these occasions, to Fort McHenry in Baltimore. The letter indicated that Dr. Conrad had just been transferred back to Drewry's Bluff from Mobile.

> Winchester Sept. 13, 1862
>
> My dear Dan,
>
> Your mother received this morning yours of the 2nd inst. from Mobile. The first news we had heard from you since the battle below Richmond.
>
> The sucesses of our army have been ever since interrupted. Gen'l Jackson's division recrossed from Maryland about Hedgesville in Beckley, two days ago, drove the enemy from Martinsburg towards Harper's Ferry; and last night followed on. The same operations have been going on below, by Walker's occupation of Leesburg, and their two wings are continually connected by a line in Maryland extending from Frederick City to Williamsport. Thus the Yankee troops in the valley are now all huddled together about the Ferry, surrounded on every side but theirs,

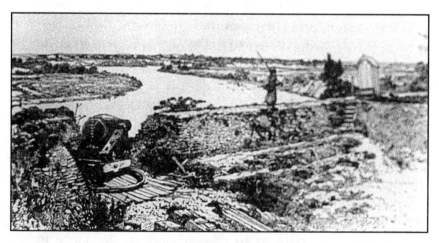

Drewry's Bluff

Fort Darling, located on the west side of the James River about seven miles south of Richmond, was manned by a Confederate heavy naval artillery detachment. Also positioned here were sharpshooters and Confederate marines.

Battles and Leaders

and we look certainly for news of their capture today or tomorrow. Their whole force is variously esti-
mated at from five to ten thousand. I suppose about
eight is the correct number, from all I have heard of
the forces at this place and the points they occupied
a week ago on the line of the B. & O. R. R. Some ap-
prehension exists that they may make an attempt to
escape by way of Winchester over to Romney &
Cumberland; and this has rec'd some credence from
a report that Gen'l Jackson sent up there last night
an order for all the wagons to be moved from here
eight miles back up the Staunton Road. They will
make no such desperate attempt, I am satisfied, but
are waiting only for a summons to surrender. My
observation of them whilst here showed they are
thoroughly cowed.

I cannot but hope that we are now in sight of the
end of this war. McClellan's whole forces cannot
stand against our forces now in Maryland, nor will
they be able to remain in Washington. The means
and credit of the Yankee government are well neigh
exhausted, and their people disgusted with the war;
to raise & bring on to the field another Northern army
seems to me almost an impossibility.

During their last occupation here the Yankees
showed themselves even more as brutal ruffians and
thieves than before, restrained by nothing but their
fear of being called on to account here after they threatened every outrage, even to extermination of our
people; arrested a number of us, held some in their
guard tents, with negroes & deserters; and sent some
off to Washington & Baltimore. All this was to induce
or force our citizens to take an oath of allegiance to
Lincoln. In this they signally failed. Afterwards they
prescribed an <u>oath of neutrality</u> during the war. Some
of our citizens seduced by the privileges & safety offered to merchandize & their property and frightened

by their threats of incarceration and gave way, and took this oath required and were of course, duly engaged in persuading others to do likewise. I made every effort in my power to prevent first the oath of allegiance and afterwards this oath of neutrality from being taken and thus incurred the special malice of the officers. They had me several times in custody at their camp, but I took the ground that as a citizen of Virginia, not in arms, they could do no more than drive me out of their lines and before I would take any oath to their government, or come under any obligation whatsoever, or recognize its authority, or right to invade the state, I would suffer their or any other consequence, even if it was to be butchered by them at the instant. Finding they could not move us from this, many put off the matter from day to day, until they finally left. Fortunately some eight or ten of our citizens were present on one or two of these occasions, and declared their determination to abide by my course. This put a stop to taking the neutrality oath. To each pass given to get out of the lines (drawn close around the town) they announced paroles and certificates of loyalty & which the recipient of the pass had to sign. And so, if you asked for any safeguard against the robbery of the soldiers, they invariably announced their conditions and in this way managed to entrap a number of our citizens. One of their generals volunteered to offer me a safeguard for my property. My reply was that I had asked for none, and would not accept it, that I was a prisoner and meant to remain so. I was also offered by the Provost Marshal a passport giving me the liberty of the whole state to go and come as I pleased upon the condition that I would merely sign a parole (without the oath) to remain neutral during the war, neither myself, or any family to give aid, comfort, & c. to their enemies. This also I promptly refused. I had never asked for or taken any pass and therefore have not been out of town for more than ten months. So far from suffering more than others (except in the mere loss of Negroes and other property) we have really fared better for maintaining this bold stand. I gave them notice that any attempt to invade my house would be met with such force as I could employ, no matter what the consequences as they evidently did not intend to proceed to extremities, no attempt or order was ever made to search or enter my house, although nearly every other house in town was searched. Some of them five or ten times. When one of their officers would come on pretense of business or curiosity, I would always meet him near the gate and stop him outside the front door.

Our horses and fowl were stolen, garden and out houses pillaged, and every kind & means of annoyance resorted to, but they never dared to carry it to the point of personal insult.

Your mother and the girls were most resolute in their holding them at bay and you would hardly imagine how well they bore themselves through all, neither health nor spirits failing for a day. Salley would sit every evening in the yard with her guitar and sing all her Southern 'Secession' songs as loudly and cheerfully as ever, whilst the Yankees were standing at the gate to listen.

Dr. William Augustus Davis

A cabinet photograph of Conrad's father-in-law. This Massachusetts native faithfully served the Confederacy.

Author's Collection

We are all well now, much relieved, of course. Holmes has been with us for a week, has now gone down with his cavalry battalion to Martinsburg. Kate and Charlie yesterday went on a visit to Miss Martie Harrison. The little boys are of great service since the servants have gone.

Your friends generally are well. We have here all the refuse of the army, some 7,000—sick, ragged, skulking, begging & c. Our stock of all kinds much reduced—but we hope soon to have free intercourse with Baltimore, which the Yankees allowed only to a favored pass; even whilst they hold the town.

Your Father

R.Y.C.[21]

Conrad returned to Virginia and reported for duty on September 17, and received the $102.70 for travelling allowances. Evidently Conrad was assigned to the Ivy Depot in Albemarle County, Virginia, near his home in Winchester.[22]

On December 30, 1862, Conrad was ordered "to proceed to Drewry's Bluff, James River and report to Captain S. S. Lee Commanding for duty to replace Surgeon A. S. Garnett, detached." Conrad reported to this large artillery fort south of Richmond on the James River on January 5.[23] There, it is assumed, he served with the naval contingent that brought the guns from the CSS *Virginia* and set up a defensive position just south of Fort Darling.

From his quarters at Drewry's Bluff, Conrad wrote the following letter to his father congratulating his father on his release from prison, for not taking the oath of loyalty to the Union and, also, inviting his father to visit him at Drewry's Bluff.

My dear Father

Of late years you have not often received letters from me, partly, from habit of not writing owing to the past and continued irregularity of the mails but chiefly from the fact that my surmises & news of the day, were contradicted the next. My want of readable information my being stationed in districts foreign and unknown and my having to act on the instant in affairs concerning myself when formally I would have consulted you by letter. I think now of going abroad to some vessel. Building my stay would be of very uncertain duration. My pay would be of first avail to us and all things considered it would be best if an opportunity offers, to accept of it. I know of none at present. There may be one in the next two months. I could have gone a year ago but did not want and do not want, wish or like. I leave you all but as now situated. I would have seen near as much of you and could have rec'd letters in England. As often, the boys are removed at great distances from me, so I do not see them sick or well. The great reason is that my pay will be valuable and greatly needed in the future for whatever be the results of the war. Poverty to all is inevitable, to those at least in Confederate lines. To all human knowledge and foresight, the War is as remote as in 1861. The exhaustion of men and means is in exact proportion and we are just as strong and capable of fighting now as the enemy are; if anything we are better off for their spirit is not so war-like and we are reduced to the alternatives of subjugation, exile, or death. I was glad to hear yesterday of your release. Can you not spare a few weeks and pay me a visit. It will not be a comfortable or exhilarating trip to look forward to but it will give you a new world of thought and reflection, something to think of; and after it is over you will be glad to have made it. I can make you comfortable here at The Bluff. You can go to the city any day and return in the evening. We are not starving as one would generally suppose, but are on short rations. The campaign appears well for us. The big fighting will not begin before May. Has the

"Currency Bill" found you with any surplus, if so send it to me to invest for you and I have endeavored to keep you and send a daily file of papers so you may be posted in the Law & Orders.

Tuesday

The above written a week ago when I heard of your being taken off with William & Mr. Boyd. I saw Mr. *Botiler* and he was to see the President and urge on him the propriety of ordering the commanding officers to cease arresting citizens on the borders as it only leads to retaliation on unoffending citizens. I hope it will be carried out. We could not hear when you were carried or for what specific cause you were arrested. Today I hear of something at home on Parole. I suppose to be released when the Morgan County prisoners are. This exchange, I will urge so soon as I hear of its being the condition of your release, but the principle must be established for all of your welfare, otherwise you will all have to leave or take the Oath. I have written to Holmes to come here as he has been nominated by Burr as captain of Commissary Dept. and I hope in a week, he will be commissioned. No answer has been sent from him. He is in Woodstock. Charley was there but I suppose has joined his regiment by this time.

Friday

I have just learned, my dear Father, of your being sent to Cumberland, in a letter from Holmes.[24]

It was during this period while Winchester was occupied by the Federal troops that the family of Dr. William Augustus Davis, Dr. Conrad's future in-laws, buried their family silver and other valuables in the family's manure pile. This hiding place was used each of the many times that Winchester was occupied. Future generations of Davises and Conrads, when eating with the family silverware, always had a glimmer of doubt about the sterility of their eating utensils.

The following letter was written after one of the many Yankee occupations of Winchester ended. In this letter from Dan's father, Robert Conrad mentions that he had recently heard news of his son from Dr. William A. Davis.

                                        Win. 24th Sept. 1862.
My dear Dan,

We were all much gratified to receive your letter this week from Richmond as the last we had previously heard was by you to the girls of the 2nd Sept. from Mobile: Doctor Davis, who came here a week ago could give an account of you.

Dr. Williams letter to his mother containing many was safely sent to her direct by Q. M. Jno. Rogers, who happened to be at our house on his way home.

We are now as uncomfortable as can well be imagined, but still happy in our relief from Yankee military rule. There are upwards of 5,000 wounded & sick soldiers in town, and every house is a hospital, with few servants and a decayed stock of provisions to be had. In one house we have badly wounded Colonel O'Neill of Alabama, and one of his lieutenants besides several sick and their nurses. A major and captain from Alabama have just left for home. Old Stephen is our factotam—but the little boys attend well to the stable & cow & cut wood—when we can get it. Wood sells for about $10 per cord. & hard to get at that; owing to the sweep the Yankees made of all our houses. Marketing & merchandise of kinds are proportionally scarce and dear. Yet, with all, we are cheerful and even rejoicing, at being once more in Dixie, with the prospect of remaining thus.

The affair over in Maryland were in truth victories—the success in each engagement being ours. But the withdrawal of our army after once entering the state is unfortunate in its immediate effects, both North & South. The cause, I apprehend, was a slight failure in the general plan, which required that the forces engaged in the capture of White at H. Ferry should have been disengaged early enough to attack McClellan on the left wing in the engagement in Middletown Valley on Sunday week last; in which event his army would certainly have been disestablished. But the surrender was not until Monday, and our auxiliary troops did not come in from the Ferry until the fight on Wednesday near Sharpsburg, on disadvantageous ground and after McClellan had been largely reinforced. The enemy then fought well and our army was much in need of rest. Therefore General Lee decided to recross the river, but against the remonstrance of Jackson, who felt sure of a complete victory if the fight was renewed next day. The enemy made not the least attempt to keep us back. Our army is now ready on the line of the Potomac, and is being rapidly reinforced by sending forward all the stragglers and other troops behind. In a day or two it will be quite fresh & larger than ever. 'Twas said that ten days rations are being cooked now at once. All the trains are ordered to the front and everything indicates an early resumption of the march northward. Some of the colonels just from the army at my house yesterday stated and seemed to believe that the purpose was to march direct to Harrisburg & thence to Cleveland in Ohio, on Lake Erie, It would be a grand coup, as the French Indians say—because it would cut off and capture the whole supply of beef cattle constantly flowing from the West to New York, as well as great quantities of grain & flour. But the enterprise, I fear is chimerical. We can go to Harrisburg, not further, with safety. Some supply of provisions and clothing for our army beyond what is found south of the Potomac is indispensable. We can not go on this way much beyond Christmas next. Our supplies, especially of beef and hogs are being rapidly used up and our troops are in a pitiably ragged condition, and hundreds barefooted. But their hearts and nerves are as stout and well strong as ever, and it is marvellous to see even poor emaciated sick boys, hardly able to lift their heads, hungry, ragged, cold, as tenacious of the cause and breathing as bold and noble a spirit as when they just took their musket in hand.

The girls are both at home—or rather at the 'cooking rooms' working from sunrise 'till dark for the sick soldiers. Your mother spends her days in the hospitals, dresses as many wounds as any surgeon, and feeds the sick. We are all well. None of our servants have been heard from. Holmes is acting as adjutant of the cavalry regiment raised by Ashby & holds no commission, but has been constantly on duty, and an acknowledged leader throughout. I hope you will come and see us soon. You might be ordered here and afterwards arrange about the transfer.

Yours

Rob. Y. Conrad[25]

Dr. Hunter McGuire, Stonewall Jackson's medical director and Conrad's childhood friend in Winchester, requested Conrad to join him on Stonewall's staff of the Second Corps of the Army of Northern Virginia. Dr. McGuire wrote to Secretary of the Navy Stephen Mallory, requesting that Dr. Conrad be transferred to the staff of Stonewall Jackson. The back of the request was endorsed by Stonewall Jackson.

Head Quarters 2nd Corps A. N. Va.

Medical Department

April 16, 1863

Sir

I respectfully request that Surgeon D. B. Conrad, C.S.N. now on duty at Chaffin's Bluff be relieved and ordered to report for temporary duty with this corps.

I am anxious to have the services of Dr. Conrad during the approaching campaign. His present position can probably be easily filled, and his field of usefulness will be extended if this temporary transfer can be granted.

Very Respectfully
Your obt Servt
Hunter McGuire
Med. Director
2nd Corps A. N. Va.

Hon. S. Mallory
    Secretary of the Navy

Among the endorsements on the back are the following:

Hd Qs 2d Corps A. N. V.
Respectfully approved
and forwarded
T. J. Jackson
M. General

and

Headquarters Army N. Va.
18 April 1863
Res. fwd and recom-
mended by order
Gen. Lee
W. H. Taylor
A. and A. G.

and

Med. Director, Staff. A.N.V.
April 17th, 1863
Respectfully returned .
The services of Dr. Conrad
with this army are very
desirable, and I hope
the transfer asked for
may be granted
L. Shields
Med. Dir. A.N.V.

and

> Resp'y referred to the secy
> the Navy
> H. L. Clay.
> A & I. G. O.
> Apl 22, '61.

and

> Office of Sec. of the Navy
> April 23d 1863
> The services of Surgeon Conrad
> C.S.N. are at this time
> indispensable, and the Navy
> Department regrets that it
> cannot assign him for the
> temporary duty (named within)
> to the Army
> By Command of Sec. of Navy
> *Jno. N. Mitchell*
> Commander in charge

and

> Resp'y returned to Genl Lee
> for his information
> By command of Sec of Navy
> H. L. Clay,
> A.A.G.
> A. & I.G.O.
> May 1, '63.[26]

Dr. Daniel B. Conrad, while at Richmond, along with his future father-in-law, Dr. William Augustus Davis, were among the large group of military physicians who organized a new professional organization in Richmond.

In August 1863 under the auspices of the surgeon general and at the invitation of the faculty of the Medical College of Virginia a large number of military surgeons from in and around Richmond met to organize an Association of the Army and Navy Surgeons of the Confederate States, which continued to the end of the war. The officers were Samuel P. Moore, president; James B. McCaw, first vice-president; Daniel Conrad, C. S. N., second vice-president, W. A. Davis, First Recording Secretary...[27]

Evidently, Dr. Conrad was then sent to Winchester because the following letter was addressed to him there. A fellow physician inquired as to what happened to a servant, John, left behind in Winchester by his sick brother.

> Charlottesville, Va.
> Sept. 3rd, 1863
>
> Dear Sir:
>
> My brother Lieutenant McIntosh informed me some time ago, that as our army was falling back by Winchester, he was forced to leave his servant John under your kind charge as he was too sick to be brought on any farther. He asked me to make some inquiries as to what had become of him, whether he was still living and whether he had fallen into Yankee hands. Will you be so kind as to let me know what has become of him. If he is alive and able to travel try and send him on to this place as I can then take charge of him and forward him to camp from here if he is in condition for it, or send him home if he needs it. And any expense or trouble you may have been put to on his account will be recompensed in such way as you desire it. Address Dr. James McIntosh—Genl. Hospt. Division No. 2—Charlottesville and you will greatly oblige by attending to this matter.
>
> Your ob't. servant
> James McIntosh
>
> To—Dr. Daniel Conrad
> Winchester[28]

The first two and a half years of the war, Dr. Conrad served with various medical units in Virginia while still assigned to the 2nd Virginia Infantry. Occasionally, he was sent to inspect and assure the efficiency of other posts around the South.

Civil War Record of Dr. William Augustus Davis

Dr. William A. Davis received his commission on November 13, 1861. Davis was promoted to surgeon on November 15, 1861.

Dr. Davis was at Chimborazo Hospital, No. 4 or "4th Division," on February 28, 1863. He signed reports as "Surgeon in charge."

On November 3, 1863, he was on the board of Consulting Surgeons for Chimborazo Hospital. On November 25, 1863, Davis was told to "hold himself in readiness to accompany the Ambulance Committee to the field in accordance with orders received from the surgeon general."

On July 12, 1864, Davis, with the Reserve Surgical Corps, received the order that he "will proceed without delay to the vicinity of the C.S. Army in the Valley and if found necessary, will establish a General Hospital at Winchester or such point as maybe found most advisable."

In the fall of 1864, Davis was in Harrisonburg, Virginia, at the General Hospital. On December 13, 1864, Davis on being relieved from the administration of General Hospital at Harrisonburg, by Surgeon B. J. Allen, was told to report again to Surgeon J. B. McCaw for assignment to duty at Chimborazo.

On March 2, 1865, he was relieved from duty at Chimborazo Hospital, Richmond, Virginia, and assigned to duty as medical purveyor. Dr. Davis was told to report to Surgeon R. Hedder Taylor, medical purveyor, Lynchburg, Virginia.

Chapter Four

Dr. Conrad Describes the Attack by the *David* against the USS *New Ironsides* at Charleston

Among the eight or 10 monographs written by Dr. Conrad, there was one in which he described the attack on the *New Ironsides* by the submarine *David,* so named to denote its small size but deadly firepower. The *David* was a craft that was not designed to be completely submerged, but was to cruise, having a very low profile with all structures below water except for a few inches of the pilot's cockpit or hatch, the top decking of the hull and the smokestack. The semisubmersible was about 50 feet long and six feet in diameter. The 1½-inch reinforced planking was covered with ¼ inch of steel plate. The *David* was not designed to shoot any projectile but carried a device or "torpedo" containing 60 pounds of black powder to detonate at the end of a pole or spar sticking out about 10 feet from the bow of the craft. This "torpedo ram" carried a crew of four and cruised at about six knots. She was commanded by Lieutenant William T. Glassell who had previously been in the United States Navy and recently released from Fort Warren for not taking the prescribed oath of allegiance. He was assisted by Assistant Engineer James H. Tomb, the Pilot J. Walker Cannon and James Stuart, the fireman.

The target for this new experimental craft was the Federal blockader, the ironclad *New Ironsides.* Conrad told about this exciting attack in the following article in the *Winchester Times* of June 7, 1893. However, Dr. Conrad made a rather serious mistake as to the date of this exploit. The attack took place on the dark moonless night of October 5, 1863.

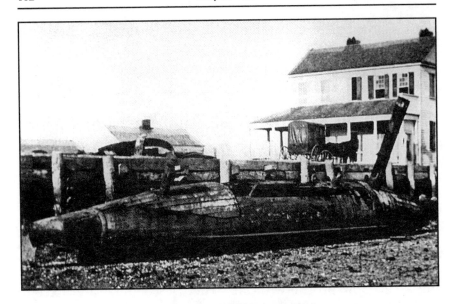

A Confederate *David* Torpedo Boat

Possibly the original, located in Charleston Harbor in 1865

Civil War Naval Chronology, 1861-1865

C. S. Receiving Ship "Dixie,"
In Charleston Harbor, S. C.,
Time—2 P.M. Nov. 10, 1864.

"Rouse up, Glassell, your number is just made from Ft. Sumpter. The signal officer reports a large 'wooden' man of war just in and anchored in the van of the blockading fleet. A stranger—has never been here before. It's cloudy, rainy, and there's no moon to-night; the best chance you've ever had. By to-morrow morning you will be a commander or in Davy Jones' locker with a gorgeous epitaph.

The above was roared into the ear of Lieut. W. T. Glassell, C. S. Navy, as he lay in his bunk on the day of his 'Torpedo Attack' in the U. S. 'New Ironsides.' He and his 'Two Volunteers' had been for many weeks sleeping 'on board' with their long torpedo boat, called the 'David,' secured along the 'Sea-ward' side of us, waiting for a dark night and a ship in the right position—and here they both were. He and they had been night owls for a month, sleeping all day, but every sundown saw them prowling around the signal station, on shore, or at the Fort, waiting and watching for just such a happening. Up at once, they begin secretly and quietly to prepare for a 'night of nervous work.' No one must even suspect the intended 'raid' lest the enemy be advised, for the U. S. 'Secret Service' fund is very large and spent with a lavish hand in the city. At sundown alone they pull over to Fort Sumter to took for themselves, to take the bearings of the 'new comer,' waiting until dark to see if and how the blockading fleet anchor for the night. Returning in the darkness they silently get up steam on board their tiny craft, so that no sound or smoke will indicate their departure.

At 9 P.M., all ready, we go down the ladder with them and step on board. It is about 30 feet long, six feet wide amidships, drawing or in depth about the same amount of water. Glassell steps into a hole aft, his head and shoulders only above deck; a night glass around his neck, a revolver in belt and a loaded shot gun alongside, the steering gear in his hands. The engineer officer, Mr. C. S. Toombs, and the fireman, Mr. J. W. Cannon, encase themselves in a similar oval hatchway amidships. To the engineer is entrusted the management of the torpedo, an oblong copper capsule filled with powder, with numerous projecting, sensitive percussion tubes. This is attached to the torpedo "spar" which swings up and down on hinges fastened to the bows. It is lifted or depressed by a well tested Manilla rope held in his hands. He also attends to the engine. The fireman looks out for the fires and boilers. Every preparation has been made in the deepest silence, and in like manner do we shake hands a "farewell" and "good luck." About

10 P.M. they disappear in the dark night, gliding noiselessly away over the misty surface of the bay. We see very shortly one signal light flash from the look out of Ft. Sumter. They have passed it and are now heading for their prey.

The next morning "Sumter" reports great commotion in the fleet about 1 (one) A.M., "signal lights and firing," and about 9 A.M. our looked for and anxiously awaited craft steams alongside of us, the torpedo gone, the spar broken off short and only two men on board, the engineer and fireman. They are warmly welcomed, and in the intervals of a voracious repast they give us their story.

The darkness had enabled them to avoid the outlying picket fleet of armed launches, which the enemy had out nightly, and they steamed straight for

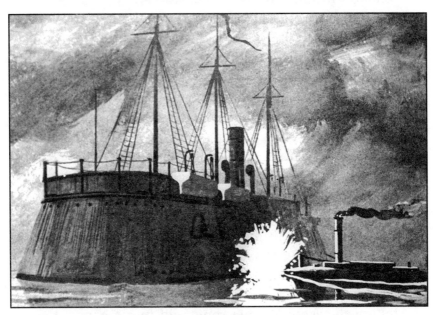

Depiction of the Attack of the Torpedo Boat *David* on the *New Ironsides* at Charleston on October 5, 1863

The *New Ironsides* was clad on both sides but not the bow or stern. She was damaged severely in this attack, but was not sunk.

Civil War Naval Chronology, 1861–1865

the motionless black mass looming in the haze. At full speed and with lowered torpedo they struck the doomed-ship under her quarter, where the officers and captain slept. A moment before Glassell had fired with his double-barrelled gun at the now thoroughly alarmed "officer of the deck, Master Howard, who, leaning over the poop railing above, had "hailed" them and fell dead on deck. There was a crash of smashed timbers, a frenzied alarm, rattles sprung and a volley of small arms. They (Glassell and his men) found themselves in the water. The collision of the two vessels and the shock of the exploding torpedo had driven their tiny boat backwards and down into the sea. She had filled. Each man struck out for himself, their cork jackets keeping them afloat. The engineer, with the instinct of his calling, kept a look out for his boat, and after a time saw it bobbing up and down in the tide-way. Out of sight of the now sinking ship, he scrambled over its side and with water up to his waist he baled away, and by a wonderful chance the fireman floated near by and hailed. He was pulled on board and the two soon cleared her of water, then relit the fires and got up steam. The attention of the enemy being fully occupied with his sinking vessel enabled them to do this safely.

Nothing could be seen or heard of Glassell. After firing his gun he had disappeared. They gave him up as lost and steamed back to the fort. By the next "flag of truce" we heard of him, a prisoner in Fort Warren. His story was that by the recoil he was thrown into the water, floated around amidst the enemy's boats a while, and not caring to be made a prisoner had swum away, and seeing a dark object made for it. It was an abandoned coal barge. Into this he climbed and there remained until sunrise revealed to him the sunken "New Ironsides" surrounded by boats. Wet, cold and famishing for both food and drink, about sunset, seeing no possible means of escape, he stood up and signaled with his coat. A boat was sent off for him and he was soon on board the "flag ship" a prisoner. He was treated as brave men treat a "daring foe," was soon exchanged and promoted to "commander"; saw hard service in the "James River Fleet" below Richmond in the spring of 1865. After the surrender he went to California where he had a brother and sister, and I understand died there not many years ago.

"All honor for this daring deed," should be his epitaph.

D. B. Conrad, M. D.,

Late Surgeon U. S. N. and C. S. N.[1]

It is not known why Conrad chose to describe this attack outside of Charleston, but history is indebted to him for this very important historical narrative.

Chapter Five

Dr. Conrad Accompanies the Confederate Raiders on the USS *Underwriter* at New Bern Bay, North Carolina

On February 23, 1864, Daniel Conrad went with J. Taylor Wood to New Bern, North Carolina, on the ultrasecret "New Bern Raid." The Confederate navy cooperated with the Confederate marine corps in a joint venture to capture one of the Federal, side-wheel gunboats operating out of New Bern and the Pamlico Sound. Commander John Taylor Wood had overall command of the operation. Conrad's friend from before the war, Lieutenant Benjamin Loyall, commandant of midshipmen on the Confederate Naval Academy schoolship *Patrick Henry*, led the Richmond contingent, consisting of 10 cutters and approximately 115 men and officers. The marine contingent was led by Colonel Lloyd J. Beall.

Dr. Conrad told about this raid to capture the four-gun side-wheel steamer, the USS *Underwriter,* in another monograph written after the war:

> In January, 1864, the Confederate naval officers on duty in Richmond, Wilmington and Charleston were aroused by a telegram from the Navy Department to detail three boats' crews of picked men and officers, who were to be fully armed, equipped and rationed for six days; they were to start at once by rail for Weldon, North Carolina, reporting on arrival to Commander J. Taylor Wood, who would give further instructions. So perfectly secret and well-guarded was our destination that not until we had

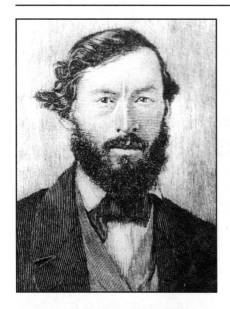

Commander John Taylor Wood

Overall commander of the joint Confederate marine and navy expedition to capture the Federal gunboat *Underwriter* at New Bern, North Carolina.

Battles and Leaders

all arrived at Kingston, North Carolina, by various railroads, did we have the slightest idea of where we were going or what was the object of the naval raid. We suspected, however, from the name of its commander, that it would be 'nervous work,' as he had a reputation for boarding, capturing and burning the enemy's gunboats on many previous occasions.

Embarking one boat after another on the waters of the Neuse, we found that there were ten of them in all, each manned by ten men and two officers, every one of whom were young, vigorous, fully alive and keen for the prospective work. Now we felt satisfied that it was going to be hand-to-hand fighting; some Federal gunboat was to be boarded and captured by us, or we were to be destroyed by it.

Sunday afternoon, February 1, 1864, about 2 o'clock, we were all quietly floating down the narrow Neuse, and the whole sunny Sabbath evening was thus passed, until at sunset we landed on a small island. After eating our supper, all hands were assembled to receive instructions. Commander Wood, in distinct and terse terms, gave orders to each boat's crew and its officers just what was expected of them, stating that the object of the expedition was to, that night, board some one of the enemy's gunboats, then supposed to be lying off the city of New Bern, now nearly sixty miles distant from where we then were by water. He said that she was to be captured without fail. Five boats were to board her on either side simultaneously, and then when in our possession we were to get up steam and cruise after other gunboats. It was a grand scheme, and was received by the older men with looks of admiration and with rapture by the young midshipmen, all of whom would have broken out into loud cheers but for the fact that the strictest silence was essential to the success of the daring undertaking.

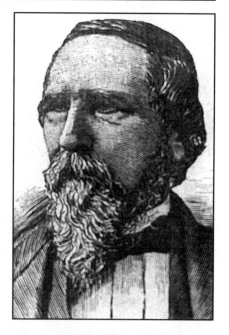

Colonel Lloyd J. Beall, CSMC
Commandant of the Confederate marines led a strike force of marines on the expedition.
Civil War Naval Chronology, 1861-1865

In concluding his talk, Commander Wood solemnly said: 'We will now pray,' and thereupon he offered up the most touching appeal to the Almighty that it had ever been my fortune to have heard. I can remember it now, after the long interval that has elapsed since then. It was the last ever heard by many a poor fellow, and deeply felt by every one.

Then embarking again, we now had the black night before us, our pilot reporting two very dangerous points where the enemy had out pickets of both cavalry and infantry. We were charged to pass these places in absolute silence, our arms not to be used unless we were fired upon, and then in that emergency we were to get out of the way with all possible speed, and pull down stream in order to surprise and capture one of the gunboats before the enemy's pickets could carry the news of our raid to them.

In one long line, in consequence of the narrowness of the stream, did we pull noiselessly down, but no interrupting pickets were discovered, and at about half past three o'clock we found ourselves upon the broad estuary of New Bern Bay. Then closing up in double column we pulled for the lights of the city, even up to and close in and around the wharves themselves, looking (but in vain) for our prey. Not a gunboat could be seen; none were there. As the day broke we hastened for shelter to a small island up stream about three miles away, where we landed upon our arrival, dragged our boats into the high grass, setting out numerous pickets at once. The remainder of us, those who were not on duty, tired and weary, threw ourselves upon the damp ground to sleep during the long hours which must necessarily intervene before we could proceed on our mission.

Shortly after sunrise we heard firing by infantry. It was quite sharp for an hour, and then died away. It turned out to be, as we afterwards learned, a futile attack by our lines under General Pickett on the works around New Bern. We were obliged to eat cold food all that day, as no fires were permissible under any cicumstances; so all we could do was to keep a sharp lookout for the enemy, go to sleep again, and wish for the night to come.

About sundown one gunboat appeared on the distant rim of the bay. She came up, anchored off the city some five miles from where we were lying, and we felt that she was our game. We began at once to calculate the number of her guns and quality of her armament, regarding her as our prize for certain.

As darkness came upon us, to our great surprise and joy, a large launch commanded by Lieutenant George W. Gift, landed under the lee of the island. He had been, by some curious circumstance, left behind, but with his customary vigor and daring impressed a pilot, and taking all the chances came down the Neuse boldly in daylight to join us in the prospective fight. His advent was a grand acquisition to our force, as he brought with him fifteen men and one howitzer.

We were now called together again, the orders to each boat's crew repeated, another prayer was offered up, and then, it being about nine o'clock, in double column we started directly for the lights of the gunboat, one of which was distinctly showing at each masthead. Pulling slowly and silently for four hours we neared her, and as her outlines became distinct, to our great surprise we were hailed man-of-war fashion, 'Boat, ahoy!' We were discovered, and, as we found out later, were expected and looked for.

This was a trying and testing moment, but Commander Wood was equal to the emergency. Jumping up, he shouted: 'Give way hard! Board at once!' The men's backs bent and straightened on the oars, and the enemy at the same moment opened upon us with small arms. The long, black sides of the gunboat, with men's heads and shoulders above them, could be distinctly seen by the line of red fire, and we realized immediately that the only place of safety for us was on board of her, for the fire was very destructive. Standing up in the boat with Commander Wood, and swaying to and fro by the rapid motion, were our marines firing from the bows, while the rest of us, with only pistol in belt, and our hands ready to grasp her black sides, were all anxious for the climb. Our coxswain, a burly, gamy Englishman, who by gesture and loud word, was encouraging the crew, steering by the tiller between his knees, his hands occupied in holding his pistols, suddenly fell forward on us dead, a ball having struck him fairly in the forehead. The rudder now having no guide, the boat swerved aside, and instead of our bows striking at the gangway, we struck the wheelhouse, so that the next boat, commanded by Lieutenant Loyall, had the deadly honor of being first on board. Leading his crew, as became his rank, duty and desire, he jumped and pulled into the gangway—now a blazing sheet of flame, and being nearsighted, having lost his glasses, stumbled and fell prone upon the deck of the gunboat, the four men who were following close up on his heels falling on top of him stone dead, killed by the enemy's bullets; each one of the unfortunate fellows having from four to six of them in his body, as we found out later. Rising, Lieutenant Loyall shook off his load of dead men, and by this time we had climbed up on the wheelhouse, Commander Wood's long legs giving him an advantage over the rest of us; I was the closest to him, but had nothing to do as yet, except to anxiously observe the progress of the hand-to-hand fighting below me. I could hear Wood's stentorian voice giving orders and encouraging the men, and then, in less than five minutes, I could distinguish a strange synchronous roar, but did not understand what it meant at first; but it soon became plain; 'She's ours,' everybody crying at the top of their voices, in order to stop the shooting, as only our own men were on their feet.

I then jumped down on the deck, and as I struck it, I slipped in the blood, and fell on my back and hands; rising immediately, I caught hold of an officer standing near me, who with an oath collared me, and I threw up his revolver just in time to make myself known. It was Lieutenant Wilkinson, who the moment he recognized me, exclaimed: 'I'm looking for you doctor; come here.' Following him a short distance in the darkness, I examined a youth who was sitting in the lap of another, and in feeling his head I felt my hand slip down between his ears, and to my horror, discovered that his head had been cleft in two by a boarding sword in the hands of some giant of the forecastle. It was Passed Midshipman Palmer Sanders, of Norfolk. Directing his body, and those of all the other killed, to be laid out aft on the quarter-deck, I went down below, looking for the wounded in the ward-room, where the lights were burning, and found half a dozen with slight shots from revolvers. After having finished my examination, a half an hour had elapsed, and when ascending to the deck again I heard the officers of the various corps reporting to Commander Wood; for immediately after the capture of the vessel, according to the orders, the engineers and firemen had been sent down to the engine-room to get up steam, and Lieutenant Loyall as executive officer, with a number of seamen had attempted to raise the anchor, cast loose the cable which secured the ship to the wharf just under the guns of Fort Stephenson, while the marines in charge of their proper officers were stationed at the gangways guarding the prisoners. The lieutenants, midshipmen and others manned the guns, of which there were six eleven-inch, as it was the intention to convert her at once into a Confederate man-o-war, and under the captured flag to go out to sea, to take and destroy as many of the vessels of the enemy as possible. But all our well-laid plans were abortive; the engineers reported the fires out, and that it would be futile to attempt to get up steam under an hour, and Lieutenant Loyall, too, after very hard work, reported it useless to spend any more time in trying to unshackle the chains, as the ship had been moored to a bouy, unless he could have hours in which to perform the work. Just at this moment, too, to bring things to a climax, the Fort under which we found that we were moored bow and stern, opened fire upon us with small arms, grape and solid shot; some of those who had escaped having reported the state of affairs on board, and this was the result.

In about fifteen minutes a solid shot or two had disabled the walking-beam, and it then became evident to all that we were in a trap, to escape from which depended on hard work and strategy. How to extricate ourselves in safety from the thus far successful expedition, was the question; but events proved that our commander was equal to the emergency.

Very calmly and clearly he directed me to remove all dead and wounded to the boats, which the several crews were now hauling to the lee side of the vessel, where they would be protected from the shots from the fort. The order was soon carried out by willing hands.

They were distributed as equally as possible. Each boat in charge of its own proper officer, and subjected under that heavy fire to that rigid discipline characteristic of the navy, manned by their regular crews, as they laid in double lines, hugging the protected lee of the ship as closely as possible, it was a splendid picture of what a body of trained men can be under cicumstances of great danger.

After an extended search through the ship's decks, above and below, we found that we had removed all the dead and wounded, and then, when the search was ended, reported to Captain Wood on the quarter-deck, where, giving his orders where the fire from the fort was very deadly and searching, he called up four lieutenants to him, to whom he gave instructions as follows two of them were to go below in the forward part of the ship, and the other two below in the afterpart, where from their respective stations they were to fire the vessel, and not to leave her until her decks were all ablaze, and then at that juncture they were to return to their proper boats and report.

The remainder of us were lying on our oars while orders for firing the ship were being carried out; and soon we saw great columns of red flames shoot upward out of the forward hatch and ward-room, upon which the four officers joined their boats. Immediately, by the glare of the burning ship, we could see the outlines of the fort with its depressed guns, and the heads and shoulders of the men manning them. As the blaze grew larger and fiercer their eyes were so dazzled and blinded that every one of our twelve boats pulled away out into the broad estuary safe and untouched. Then we all realized fully our adroit and successful escape.

Some years after the affair I met one of the Federal officers who was in the fort at the time, and he told me that they were not only completely blinded by the flames, which prevented them from seeing us, but were also stampeded by the knowledge of the fact that there were several tons of powder in the magazine of the vessel, which when exploded would probably blow the fort to pieces; so, naturally, they did not remain very long after they were aware that the ship had been fired. This all occurred as we had expected. We in our boats, at a safe distance of more than half a mile, saw the 'Underwriter' blow up, and distinctly heard the report of the explosion, but those at the fort, a very short distance from the ship, sought a safe refuge, luckily for them.

Fortunately there was no casualties at this stage of the expedition. I boarded boat after boat in my capacity as surgeon, attending to the requirements of those who demanded immediate aid, and I witnessed many amusing scenes; for among the prisoners were some old men-of-war's men, former shipmates of mine in the Federal navy years before, and of the other officers also. Their minds were greatly relieved when I made known to them who their captors were, and that their old surgeon and other officers were present, and as a natural consequence they would be treated well.

Continuing to pull for the remainder of the night, we sought and found by the aid of our pilot, a safe and narrow creek, up which we ascended, and at sunrise hauled our boats up on a beach, there we carefully lifted out our wounded men, placed them under the shade of trees in the grass, and made them as comfortable as possible under the circumstances. Then we laid out the dead, and after carefully washing and dressing them, as soon as we had partaken of our breakfast, of which we were in so much need, all hands were called, a long pit was dug in the sand, funeral services were held, the men buried and each grave marked.

We remained there all that day recuperating, and when night came again embarked on our return trip all through that night and the four succeeding ones, we cautiously pulled up the rapid Neuse, doing most of our work in the darkness, until when nearing Kingston we could with impunity pull in daylight.

Arriving at Kingston, the boats were dragged up the hill to the long train of gondola cars which had been waiting for us, and then was presented an exhibition of sailors' ingenuity. The boats were placed upright on an even keel lengthwise on the flat cars, and so securely lashed by ropes that the officers, men, even the wounded, seated and laid in them as if on the water, comfortably and safely made the long journey of a day and two nights to Petersburg. Arriving, the boats were unshipped into the Appomattox River, and the entire party floated down it to City Point where it debouches into the James. It was contemplated that when City Point was reached to make a dash at any one Federal gunboat, should there be the slightest prospect of success; but learning from our scouts, on our arrival after dark, that the gunboats and transports at anchor there equalled the number of our own boats at least, we had to abandon our ideas of trying to make a capture, and were compelled to hug the opposite banks very closely, where the river is nearly four miles wide, and in that manner slip up the James pulling hard against the current. By the next evening we arrived, without any further adventure, at Drury's Bluff, where we disembarked; our boats shown as mementoes of the searching fire we had been subjected to—for they all were perforated by many minnie balls, the white wooden plugs inserted into the holes averaging fourteen to each boat engaged; they were all shot into them from stem to stern lengthwise.

Among the many incidents that occurred on the trip there were two which left a lasting impression on my mind, and to this day they are as vivid as if they had happened yesterday. As we were stepping into the boats at the island that night, the lights of the gunboat plainly visible from the spot on which we stood, a bloody, serious action inevitable, several of the midshipmen, youth-like, were gaily chatting about what they intended to do—joyous and confident, and choosing each other for mates to fight together shoulder to shoulder—when one of them who stood near me in the darkness made the remark, as a conclusion as we were taking our places in the boats: 'I wonder, boys, how many of us will be up in those stars by tomorrow morning?' This rather jarred on the ears of we older ones, and looking around to see who it was that had spoken, I recognized the bright and handsome Palmer Sanders. Poor fellow, he was the only one who took his flight, though many of the others were severely wounded.

On our route down to Kingston by rail we were obliged to make frequent stops for wood and water, and at every station the young midshipmen swarmed into the depots and houses, full of their fun and deviltry, making friends of the many pretty girls gathered there, who asked all manner of questions as to this strange sight of boats on cars filled with men in uniform new to them.

The young gentlemen explained very glibly what they were going to do—'to board, capture and destroy as many of the enemy's gunboats as possible.' 'Well, when you return,' replied the girls, 'be sure that you bring us some relics -flags, &c.' 'Yes, yes; we'll do it,' answered the boys. 'But what will you give us in exchange?' 'Why, only thanks, of course.' 'That won't do. Give us a kiss for each flag—will you?'

With blushes and much confusion, the girls consented, and in a few moments we were off and away on our journey again. On the return trip the young men, never for an instant forgetting the bargain they had made, manufactured several miniature flags. We old ones purposely stopped at all the stations we had made coming down in order to see the fun. The young ladies were called out at each place, and after the dead were lamented, the wounded in the cars cared for, then the midshipmen brought out their flags, recalled the promises made to them, and demanded their redemption. Immediately there commenced a lively outburst of laughter and denials, a skirmish, followed by a slight resistence, and the whole bevy were kissed _seriatim_ by the midshipmen, and but for the whistle of train warning them away, they would have continued indefinitely."[1]

The Confederate Congress unanimously passed a joint resolution on February 15, 1864, praising Commander Wood and his commmand for their various exploits, including the capture of the _Underwriter_.[2] Dr. Conrad once again showed his bravery under fire and dedication to the Southern cause.

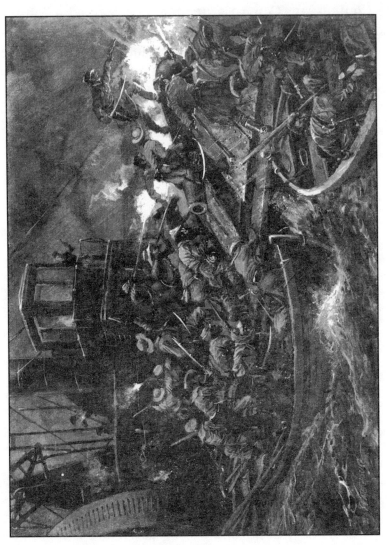

USS *Underwriter*

A painting of the storming of the *Underwriter*. The operation took place on a dark and moonless night which concealed the approach of the boarding boats.

By permission of Colonel Charles Waterhouse

Chapter Six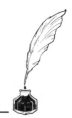

Dr. Daniel Conrad aboard the CSS *Tennessee* and the Battle of Mobile Bay

In April 1864, Conrad was ordered to Mobile as fleet surgeon with Admiral Franklin Buchanan. The Confederate fleet consisted of the ironclad ram *Tennessee* and the gunboats *Morgan*, *Gaines*, and *Selma* which had been resting at anchor to the north of Fort Morgan. Dr. Conrad, as fleet surgeon, lived on board the *Tennessee* until the action of August 5, the Battle of Mobile Bay. Into this bay would sail a large Federal fleet.

Thirty years after the Battle of Mobile Bay, Daniel Conrad wrote in the patriotic publication, *Blue and Gray*, about the construction and preparations taken by the Confederates to ready the *Tennessee* for the upcoming action to take place in a few days.

> Thirty years ago this month (August 1894) a memorable action was fought in Mobile Bay, between ironclads of different type, design, and armament; one with a shield and rifled guns, the other with turrets and Dahlgrens (smooth-bores). Many men are now living in New Orleans and Mobile who participated in or saw this conflict; there are many sons and daughters of the men living who have heard of it at the fireside. There are many others who have never heard of the fight, fought so near their homes. For these, too, I write.
>
> The Bay of Mobile was of infinite use and importance to the Confederates, who guarded and held it

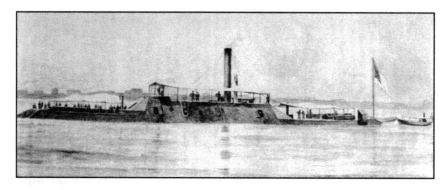

CSS *Tennessee*

A drawing by F. Muller of the ironclad CSS *Tennessee* with a Confederate flag flying from the stern. The ironclad was not rigged for battle because the awnings are deployed.

R. Thomas Campbell, *Southern Thunder*

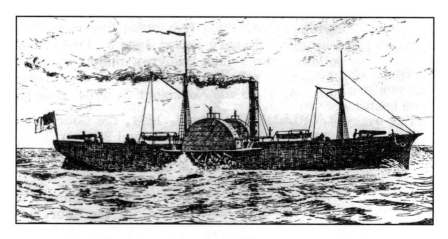

CSS *Gaines*

A side-wheel steamer of 863 tonnage. At Mobile Bay, she had trouble with her steering after taking a beating from the USS *Hartford* and *Richmond*. Her captain soon found she was sinking so he ran the *Gaines* aground near Fort Morgan.

Donald G. Shomette, *Shipwrecks of the Civil War*

by two forts, Morgan and Gaines, at its entrance. By holding it they held safe the city of Mobile from attack by water; it could only be captured by a combined army and navy attack, so it was a safe depot for blockade-runners, easy to go out of and enter, and if it was such to the Confederates, how much greater was it to the Federals? For they were compelled to keep their large blockade fleet outside, exposed to all the storms of the gulf. They could only be victualed and watered by going away, one at a time, to Pensacola, their only port; their sick had to be transported to the same place, and the wear and tear both to vessels and crews was fearful, as a constant, vigilant, and never-ceasing watch, both by officers and men, had to be kept up, day and night, year in and year out. The officers were in three watches, the men in two, guarding themselves against night attacks by torpedo boats or assault by the Confederate gunboats, and seeing that no vessel came out and that none went in. All this had to be endured, or the bay captured and held by the fleet. This was finally determined on by Farragut, and he only awaited the arrival of ironclads to make sure his end. Finding this plan determined on, the Confederates bestirred themselves. At the hamlet of Selma, on the river above, they built one ironclad, on the plan of the *Merrimac*, their resources being exhausted to do even this. Slowly the wooden structure approached completion, then more slowly was it ironed all over above the waterline, then towed down to Mobile, where it was equipped with eight-inch rifle-guns.

Then, when officers and men, provisions and water had been taken on board, all ready for action, she started down the bay, nearly thirty miles, to go outside in rough water and attack the enemy's wooden fleet before the ironclads arrived; when, on arriving at the bar of sand caused by Dog Run emptying into the bay, it was found that the bar had shoaled to such an extent that the ironclad, now christened the *Tennessee,* drew three feet more water than there was under her. The only expedient that offered itself, which was safe and speedy, was to build of huge square timbers two enormous air-tight tanks, each as high as a two-story house. They were to be towed alongside of the ram and sunk to the water's edge by opening the valves, then all lashed together securely, making one vessel, as it were, of them; the water was pumped out of these tanks, and the air entering, they, by their buoyancy, lifted the huge ship clear of the bottom, then steam tugs towed her over the bar. This was done in May 1864; it should have been so many months before, for these so-called 'camels' were finished in March. But on their arrival off Mobile they were burned by Federal emissaries, who were paid well for their daring deed.

Right here we may interrupt our story to say that the secret service fund was well spent by Admiral Farragut, for we were delayed several months in building two more 'camels,' and by that time his ironclads were built and on their way to him. I must mention the desertion of five men the day after the destruction of the camels; they had been working on our ironclad, and furnished him with all details of her construction, all her weak points, of the character of her engines, the calibre of her armament, of all of which information he availed himself when the eventful day of action came. In addition to this, they were to be received into the Federal service if they destroyed these camels. These large bribes were offered for the reason that the fleet lying outside of Fort Morgan were solely wooden ships, and could not cope with nor resist the attack of our ironclad, and the Federal ironclads had not yet arrived. Finally, one June day we were towed over the bar down the bay; then, casting loose, we steamed out to attack the Federal fleet. Reaching the passage between the two forts, we encountered rough water and found that, owing to want of buoyancy, we were in great danger of being water-logged and sunk by the amount of water that swept inboard. The ram lay deep in the water, solid and motionless as a cast-iron platform or raft, and every sea tumbling over her came inboard in such masses that the fires in the engine-room were nearly put out and the empty vessel itself filled with salt water. So discomfited, we put back under the fort, in smooth water, and all thought of attacking the fleet outside was dismissed. Then the defects, which this short cruise of ten hours had developed, were looked into. Our engines had been taken from an old river boat; they were weak and old, and could only force us through the water about two miles an hour. They could not be strengthened by any method. The rudder-chains, by which the ship was steered, were found to be exposed to the enemy's shot, being in their whole length outside the iron deck; they were covered over by a slight coating of iron rail. The capacity of the ram inboard to accommodate her crew was fearfully deficient; all officers and men, when the weather admitted slept outside on top of the iron shield and decks, but in rainy times it was awful to endure such close quarters at night; but we bore it June and July, under the sloping sides of the shield, in shape like the roof of a square house, about twelve feet in height and forty-eight in length. On July 26th, Admiral Buchanan and staff came aboard; for, from his information, a fierce fight was imminent, when, on the 1st of August, 1864, we saw a decided increase in the Federal fleet, which was then listlessly at anchor outside of Fort Morgan, in the Gulf of Mexico..."[1]

Conrad told about this battle at Mobile Bay in a paper published in the *Southern Historical Society Papers.* Conrad mistakenly remembers the captain of the *Tennessee* being named Johnson instead of James D. Johnston. It will hereafter be corrected.

...We had been lying idly in Mobile Bay for many months, on board the ironclad ram *Tennessee*, whose fighting deck differed materially from that of the Federal monitors.

It resembled the inside of the hip-roof of a house, rather than the 'cheese-box' of Ericsson's *Monitor*. On the 1st of August, 1864, we saw a decided increase in the Federal fleet, which was then listlessly at anchor outside of Fort Morgan, in the Gulf of Mexico, consisting of eight or ten wooden frigates, all stripped to a 'girt line' and clean for action; their topmasts sent down on deck and devoid of everything that seemed like extra rigging. They appeared like 'prize fighters' ready for the 'ring.' Then we knew that trouble was ahead, and wondered to ourselves why they did not enter the bay any day. On the 3rd of August we noticed another accretion to the already formidable fleet; this was four strange-looking, long, black monsters—the new ironclads—and they were what the Federals had been so anxiously waiting for. At the distance of four miles their lengthy dark lines could only be distinguished from the sea on which they sat motionless, by the continuous volume of thick smoke issuing from their low smoke-stacks, which appeared to come out of the ocean itself. These curious-looking crafts made their advent on the evening of the 4th of August, and then we knew that the 'guage of battle' was offered.

We had been very uncomfortable for many weeks in our berths on board the *Tennessee*, in consequence of the prevailing heavy rains wetting the decks, and the terrible moist, hot atmosphere, simulating that oppressiveness which precedes a tornado. It was, therefore, impossible to sleep inside; besides, from the want of properly-cooked food, and the continuous wetting of the decks at night, the officers and the men were rendered desperate. We knew that the impending action would soon be determined one way or the other, and every one looked forward to it with a positive feeling of relief.

I had been sleeping on the deck of the admiral's cabin for two or three nights, when at daybreak, on the 5th of August, the old 'quartermaster' came down the ladder, rousing us up with his gruff voice, saying: 'Admiral, the officer of the deck bids me report that the enemy's fleet is under way.' Jumping up, still half asleep, we came on deck, and sure enough, there was the enemy heading for the 'passage' past the fort. The grand old admiral, of sixty years, with his countenance rigid and stern, showing a determination for battle in every line, then gave his only order;

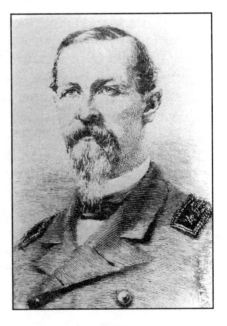

Commander James D. Johnston, CSN

He surrendered the *Tennessee* when its exterior steering chain was severed at Mobile Bay in August of 1864.

Battles and Leaders

'Get under way, Captain Johnston; head for the leading vessel of the enemy, and fight each one as they pass us.'

The fort and fleet, by this time, had opened fire, and the *Tennessee* replied, standing close in, and meeting the foremost as they came up. We could could see two long lines of men-of-war; the innermost was composed of the four monitors, and the outer of the ten wooden frigates, all engaging the fort and fleet. Just at that moment we expected the monitors to open fire upon us, there was a halt in the progress of the enemy's fleet. We observed that one of the monitors was apparently at a standstill; she 'laid to' for a moment, seemed to reel, then slowly disappear into the gulf. Immediately immense bubbles of steam, as large as cauldrons, rose to the surface of the water, and only eight human beings could be seen in the turmoil. Boats were sent to their rescue, both from the fort and fleet, and they were saved. Thus the monitor *Tecumseh*, at the commencement of the fight, struck by a torpedo, went to her fate at the bottom of the gulf, where she still lies. Sunk with her was her chivalric commander T. A. M. Craven; the pilot, an engineer, and two seamen were the only picked up by the Federal boats, and they were on duty in the turret. The pilot, whom I sometime afterward conversed with at Pensacola, on the subject, told me that when the vessel careened, so that water began to run into the mouth of the turret, he and Captain Craven were on the ladder together, the captain on the top step, with the way open for his easy and honorable escape; the pilot said: 'Go ahead, captain!' 'No, sir,' replied Craven; 'after you, pilot! I leave my ship last!' Upon this the pilot sprung up, and the gallant Craven went down, sucked under in the vortex, thus sacrificing himself through a chivalric sense of duty.

There was a dead silence on board the *Tennessee*; the men peered through the portholes at the awful catastrophe, and spoke to each other only in low whispers; for they knew that the same fate was, probably, awaiting us, for we were then directly over the torpedo bed, and, shut up tightly as we were in our iron capsule, in another moment it might prove our coffin.

At this juncture the enemy's leading vessel 'backed water' and steered on one side, which arrested the progress of the whole squadron. But at this supreme moment the second vessel, Admiral [David] Farragut's flagship, the *Hartford*, forged ahead, and Farragut, showing the nerve and determination of the officer and the man, gave the order: 'Damn the torpedoes! Go ahead!' And away he went, crushing through their bed to victory and renown. Some of the officers told me afterwards that they could hear the torpedoes snapping under the bottoms of their ships, and that they expected every moment to be blown into high air.

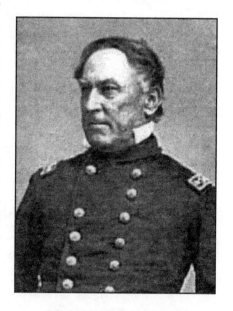

Admiral David Farragut, USN

The Southern-born admiral led the Federal naval force in its attempt to defeat the Confederate forces at Mobile Bay.

The slightest delay at that time on the part of Farragut, subjected as he was to the terrible fire of the fort and the fleet, would have been disaster, defeat, and the probable loss of his entire squadron, but he proved to be the mean for the emergency.

We, in the *Tennessee*, advancing slowly, at the rate of about two miles an hour, met the leading vessels of the enemy as they passed, and fought them face to face; but their fire was so destructive, continuous

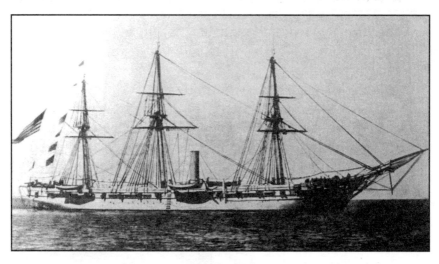

USS *Hartford*

Flagship of the Federal fleet. It was from the riggings of this ship that Farragut led the fight against the *Tennessee.*

Civil War Naval Chronology, 1861-1865

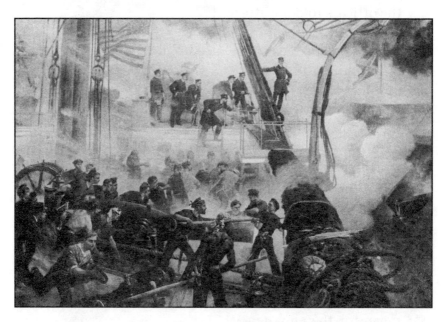

Painting of *An August Morning with Farragut* by William H. Overend

The painting illustrates Admiral Farragut lashed to the mizzen rigging, the proximity of the *Tennessee,* and some of the 40 to 50 dents in her armor.

Naval Historical Center

and severe that after we emerged from it there was nothing left standing as large as your little finger. Everything had been shot away, smokestacks, staunchions, boat davits, and in fact, fore and aft, our deck had been swept absolutely clean. A few of our men were slightly wounded, and when the last vessel had passed us and been fought in turn, we had been in action more than an hour and a half; and then the enemy's fleet, somewhat disabled, of course, kept on up the bay, and anchored about four miles away—so ended the first part of the fight. Farragut had already won half the battle; he had passed the fort and fleet, and had ten wooden vessels and three monitors left in good fighting trim.

Neither the officers or men of either fleet had as yet been to breakfast, and the order was given, 'Go to breakfast!' For us on the *Tennessee* to eat below was simply impossible, on account of the heat and humidity. The heat below was terrific; intense thirst universally prevailed. The men rushed to the scuttle-butts, or water tanks, and drank greedily. Soon 'hard tack' and coffee were furnished, the men all eating standing, creeping out of the ports on the afterdeck to get a little fresh air, the officers going to the upper deck.

Admiral Buchanan, grim, silent and rigid with prospective fighting, was 'stumping' up and down the deck, lame from a wound received in his first engagement in the *Merrimac*, and in about fifteen minutes we observed that instead of heading for the safe lee of the fort, our iron prow was pointed for the enemy's fleet. Suppressed exclamations were beginning to be heard from the officers and crew; 'The old admiral has not had his fight out yet; he is heading for that big fleet; he will get his fill of it up there!'

Slowly and gradually this fact became apparent to us, and I, being on his staff and in close association with him, ventured to ask him: 'Are you going into that fleet, admiral?' 'I am, sir!' was his reply. Without intending to be hear by him I said to an officer standing near me: 'Well, we'll never come out of there whole!' But Buchanan had heard my remark, and turning around said sharply: 'That's my lookout, sir!' And now began the second part of the fight.

I may as well explain here why he did this much-criticised and desperate deed of daring. He told me his reasons long afterwards as follows: He had only had six hours' coal on board, and he intended to expend that in fighting. He did not mean to be trapped like a rat in a hole, and made to surrender without a struggle! Then he meant to go to the lee of the fort and assist General Payne in the defense of the place. This calculation was unluckily prevented by the shooting away of the rudder chains of the *Tennessee* in this second engagement.

As we approached the enemy's fleet one after another of Farragut's ten wooden frigates swept out in a wide circle, and by the time we reached the point where the monitors were, a huge leading frigate was coming at the rate of ten miles an hour, a column of white foam formed of the dead water piled in front of its bows many feet high. Heavy cannonading from the monitors was going on at this time, when the leading wooden vessel came rapidly bearing down on us, bent on the destruction of the formidable ram, which we on board of the *Tennessee* fully realized as the supreme moment of the test of our strength. We had escaped from the torpedo bed safe and on top, and were now to take our chances of being run under by the heavy wooden frigates that were fast nearing us. Each vessel had her bows heavily ironed for the purpose of cutting down and sinking the *Tennessee*, as such were the orders of Admiral Farragut.

Captain Johnston, in the pilothouse, gave the word to officers and men: 'Steady yourselves when she strikes. Stand by and be ready!' Not a word was heard on the deck, under its shelving roof, where the officers and men, standing by their guns, silent and rigid, awaited their fate. Captain Johnston then shouted out: 'We are all right! They can never run us under now!' As he spoke the leading vessel had struck against our 'overhang' with tremendous impact; had shivered its iron prow in the clash, but only succeeded in whirling the *Tennessee* around, as if it were swung on a pivot.

I was sitting on the combing of the hatch, having nothing to do as yet, a close observer, as each vessel in turn struck us. At the moment of impact they slid alongside of us, and our black wales came in contact. At a distance of ten feet they poured their broadsides of twenty eleven-inch guns into us. This continued for more than an hour, and as each vessel 'rammed' the *Tennessee* and slid alongside, they followed, discharging their broadsides fast and furious, so that the noise was one continuous, deafening roar. You could only hear voices when spoken close to the ear, and the reverberation was so great that bleeding at the nose was not infrequent.

Soon the wounded began to pour down to me. Stripped to their waists, the white skins of men exhibited curious dark-blue elevations and hard spots. Cutting down to these, I found that unburnt cubes of cannon powder, that had poured into the ports, had perforated the flesh and made these great blue ridges under the skin. Their sufferings were very severe, for it was as if they had been shot with red-hot bullets; but no serious effects followed.

Now all the wooden vessels, disabled and their prows broken off, anchored in succession some half a mile away. Then Admiral Farragut signaled to the

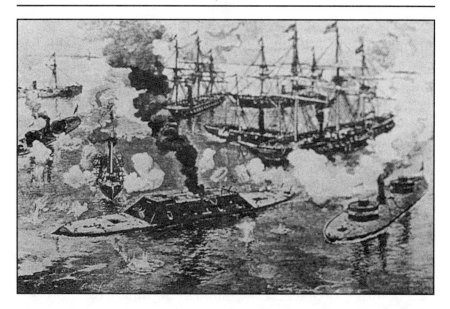

The *Tennessee* surrounded by the *Hartford* and her supporting cast of gunboats.

Civil War Naval Chronology, 1861–1865

monitors: 'Destroy the Ram!' Soon these three grim monsters, at thirty yards distance, took their position on each quarter of the *Tennessee*, as she had laid nearly motionless, her rudder having been shot away with grape in the fight. We knew that were hopelessly disabled, and that victory was impossible, as all we could do was to move around very slowly in a circle, and the only chance left to us was to crawl under the shelter of Fort Morgan.

For an hour and a half the monitors pounded us with solid shot, fired with a charge of sixty pounds of powder from their eleven-inch guns, determined to crush in the shield of the *Tennessee*, as thirty pounds of powder was the regulation amount. In the midst of this continuous pounding, the port-shutter of one of our guns was jammed by a shot, so that it could neither open nor shut, making it impossible to work the piece. The admiral then sent for some of the firemen from below, to drive the bolt outward.

Four men came up, and two of them holding the bolt back, the others struck it with sledgehammers. While they were thus standing there, suddenly there was a dull sounding impact, and at the same instant the men whose backs were against the shield were split in pieces. I saw their limbs and chests, severed and mangled, scattered about the deck, their hearts lying near their bodies. All of the gun's crew and the admiral were covered from head to foot with blood, flesh and viscera. I thought at first that the admiral was mortally wounded. The fragments and members of the dead men were shoveled up, put in buckets and hammocks, and struck below.

Engineer Rogers, of the wounded, had a pistol ball through his shoulder. 'How in the world did you manage to get this?' I asked him. He replied: 'Why, I was off watch and had nothing to do, so while the *Hartford* was lying alongside of us a Yankee cursed me through the porthole and I jabbed him with my bayonet in the body, and his comrade shot me with his revolver.' Cutting the ball out, I proposed to give him morphine, as he was suffering terribly, but he said: 'None of that for me, doctor. When we go down I want to be up and take my chances of getting out of some porthole.' Another man was wounded in the ear when fighting in the same manner as the engineer, but he always declared he got even by the use of his bayonet. I merely mention these facts to show how close the fighting was, when men could kill or wound each other through the portholes of their respective vessels.

While attending the engineer, an aide came down the ladder in great haste and said: 'Doctor, the admiral is wounded!' 'Well, bring him below,' I replied. 'I can't do it,' he answered; 'I haven't time. I am carrying orders for Captain Johnston.' So up I went;

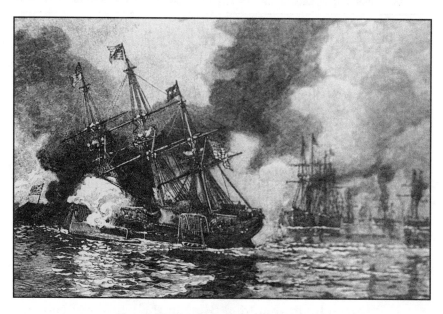

The *Hartford* Colliding with the *Tennessee*

During those close encounters, some crewmen resorted to pistols and muskets.

Battles and Leaders

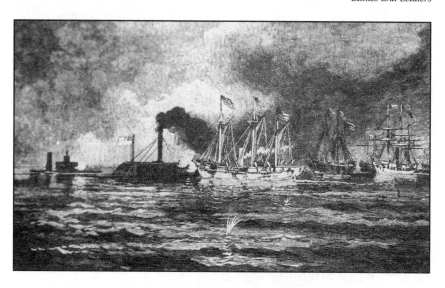

The *Monongahela* Ramming the *Tennessee*

This naval battle that started at 6:47 A.M. ended by ten o'clock.

Battles and Leaders

asked some officer whom I saw: 'Where is the admiral?' 'Don't know,' he replied. 'We are all at work loading and firing. Got too much to do to think of anything else.' Then I looked for the gallant commander myself, and, lying curled up under the sharp angle of the roof, I discovered the old white-haired man. He was grim, silent, and uttered no sound in his great pain. I went up to him and asked: 'Admiral, are you badly hurt?' 'Don't know,' he replied; but I saw one of his legs crushed up under his body, and, as I could get no help, raised him up with great caution and, clasping his arms around my neck, carried him on my back down the ladder to the cockpit, his broken leg slapping against me as I moved slowly along. After I had applied a temporary bandage he sat up on the deck and received reports from Captain Johnston regarding the progress of the fight. Captain Johnston soon came down in person, and the admiral greeted him with: 'Well, Johnston, they have got me again. You'll have to look out for her now; it is your fight.' 'All right,' answered the captain; 'I'll do the best I know how.'

In the course of half an hour Captain Johnston again made his appearance below and reported to the admiral that all the frigates had 'hauled off,' but that the three monitors had taken position on our quarters. He added that we could not bring a gun to bear, and that the enemy's solid shot were gradually smashing in the shield, and that not having been able to fire for thirty minutes, the men were fast becoming demoralized from sheer inactivity, and that from the smashing of the shield, they were seeking shelter, which showed their condition mentally. 'Well, Johnson,' said the admiral at this precarious juncture, 'Fight to the last! Then to save these brave men, when there is no longer any hope, surrender.'

In twenty minutes more the firing ceased, Captain Johnston having bravely gone up alone on the exposed roof with a handkerchief on a boarding dike, and the surrender was effected. Then we immediatley carried all our wounded upon the roof into the fresh air, which they so much needed.

From that elevated place I witnessed the rush of the petty officers and the men of the monitor, which was nearest to us, to board the captured ship to procure relics and newspaper renown. Two creatures dressed in blue shirts, begrimed and black with powder, rushed up to the wounded admiral and demanded his sword! His aide refused peremptorily, whereupon one of them stooped as if to take it anyhow, upon which Aide Forrest warned him not to touch it, as it would only be given to Admiral Farragut, or his authorized representative. Still the man attempted to seize it, whereupon Forrest knocked him off the shield to the deck below. At this critical moment, when a fight was imminent, I saw a boat nearing, flying a captain's pennant, and running down as it came alongside, I recognized an old shipmate, Captain LeRoy. I hurriedly explained to him our position, whereupon he mounted the shield, and assuming command, he arrested the obnoxious man, and sent him under guard to his boat.

The sword was then given to Captain Giraud by Admiral Buchanan, to be carried to Admiral Farragut. Our flag, smoke-stained and torn, was seized by the other man, and hastily concealed in his shirt bosom. He was brought before Captain LeRoy, and amidst the laughter and jeers of his companions, was compelled to draw it forth from its hiding place, and it was sent on board the flagship. These two heroes were said to be the correspondents of some New York and Chicago newspapers.

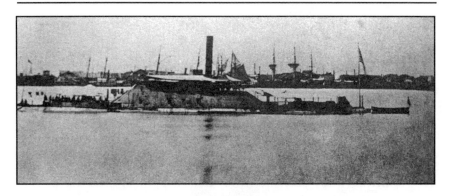

CSS *Tennessee*

This photograph of the *Tennessee* was taken while it remained at Mobile Bay in 1865, after being captured with the Federal flag flying at the stern. Notice the awnings shielding the decks.

Civil War Naval Chronology, 1861-1865

Captain LeRoy, who was an old friend, immediately had private supplies brought, and did everything in his power to aid his former shipmate, the wounded admiral. He brought a kind message from Admiral Farragut, in which the latter expressed regret to hear of Admiral Buchanan's wound, and offered to do anything in his power, and wishing to know what he desired. This was accepted by Admiral Buchanan in the same kind spirit in which it was given, and, as one of his staff officers, I was sent on board the *Hartford* with the reply: 'That appreciating the kind message, he had only to ask that his fleet-surgeon and his aids might be allowed to accompany him wherever he might be sent, until his recovery from his wound.' Boarding the *Hartford*, by Captain LeRoy's steam-launch, ascending by the man-rope, I mounted the hammock netting as the whole starboard side, amidship, and the gangway had been carried away, as I was afterwards told, by one of their own frigates having collided with the *Hartford*, after ramming the *Tennessee*. From the hammock-nettings the scene was one of carnage and devastation. The spar-deck was crowded and littered with broken gun-cartridges, shattered boats, disabled guns, and a long line of grim corpses dressed in blue, lying side by side. The officers accompanying me told me that those men—two whole gun's crews—were all killed by splinters; and pointing with his hand to a piece of weather-boarding ten feet long and four inches wide, I received my first and vivid idea of what a splinter was, or what was meant by a splinter. Descending, we threaded our way, and ascending the poop, where all of the officers were standing, I was taken up and introduced to Admiral Farragut, whom I found a very quiet, unassuming man, and not in the least flurried by his great victory. In the kindest manner he inquired regarding the severity of the admiral's wound, and then gave the necessary orders to carry out Admiral Buchanan's request.

We then thought that the admiral's leg would have to be amputated that evening or the next morning. In speaking to the admiral about his chances for recovery and the proposed amputation, he replied: 'I have nothing to do with it. It is your leg now; do your best.' It was this spirit of firmness and equanimity which not only saved Admiral Buchanan's life, but ultimately his leg also. He was carried on board of Captain James E. Jouett's ship, the *Metacomet*, which was temporaily converted into a hospital. We remained on board that night and were cared for in every kind way by Captain Jouett, to whom Admiral Buchanan always expressed himself as deeply indebted.

The next morning, at my suggestion, a flag of truce was sent to General Page, commanding Fort Morgan, representing our condition, sending the names of our dead, wounded, and the great number of Federals dead and wounded on board, and asked, in the name of humanity, to be allowed to pass the fort and convey all of them to the large naval hospital at Pensacola, where they all could receive the same treatment. To this question General Page promptly responded, and we passed out, and in eight hours were all safely housed in the ample hospital, where we were treated by old navy friends in the warmest and kindest manner. Medical Director Turner was in charge, and we remained there until December, when Admiral Buchanan being able to hobble around on crutches, was conveyed to Fort Warren with his aide, and I was sent back to Mobile in Captain Jouett's ship, under flag of truce.

Daily with the admiral in hospital at Pensacola for four months, he explained his whole plan of action to me of that second fight in Mobile Bay as follows: 'I did not expect to do the passing vessels any serious injury; the guns of Fort Morgan were thought capable of doing that. I expected that the monitors would then and there surround me, and pound the shield in; but when all the Federal vessels had passed up and anchored four miles away, then I saw that long siege was intended by the army and navy, which with its numerous transports at anchor under Pelican Island, were debarking nearly 10,000 infantry. I determined then, having the example before me of the blowing up of the *Merrimac* in the James River by our own officers, without a fight, and by being caught in such a trap, I determined, by an unexpected dash into the fleet, to attack and do it all the damage in my power; to expend all my ammunition and what little coal I had on board, only six hours' steaming, and then, having done all I could with what resources I had, to retire under the guns of the fort, and being without motive power, there to lay and assist in repulsing the attacks and assaults on the fort.'

The unexpectedness of the second attack is well illustrated by Admiral Farragut's remark at the time: 'After having anchored, all hands were piped to breakfast, when the officer on duty on the deck of the *Hartford* seeing the ram slowly heading up the bay for the Federal fleet, reported the fact to Admiral Farragut while he was taking his breakfast. "What! is that so?" he inquired. "Just like Buchanan's audacity. Signal to all frigates to get immediately under way and run the ram under, and to the monitors to attack at once."'

The greatest injury done to the *Tennessee* was by the *Chickasaw*, commanded by Captain G. H. Perkins. Our pilot, in pointing it out to Captain Johnston, said: 'That d——d iron clad is hanging to us like a dog, and has smashed our shield already. Fight him! Sink him if you can!' The *Chickasaw* really captured the *Tennessee*.

Admiral Buchanan was in form and physique one out of many. Upright in his carriage, he walked like a game-cock, though halting in his gait in later years in consequence of having received a minnie ball in his right thigh when commanding the *Merrimac* in the first ironclad fight in the world. It was while he stood on the deck, after sinking the *Congress*, that he was shot by some Federal infantry on the shore, and from 1864 to his death in 1871, he was very lame in both legs—the left one particularly—which was terribly shattered in the fight when in the *Tennessee*. He always complained of his bad luck in his two great actions; in the first he was struck down at the moment of victory, and in the last at the moment of defeat. At sixty-two years he was a strikingly handsome old man; clean shaved, ruddy complexion, with a very healthy hue, for he was always remarkably temperate in all his habits; he had a high forehead, fringed with snow-white hair; thin close lips, steel-blue eyes, and projecting conspicuously was that remarkable feature which impressed every one and marked him as one of a thousand, his wonderful aquiline nose, high, thin and perfect in all its outlines. When full of fight he had a peculiarity of drawing down the corners of his mouth until the thin line between his lips performed a perfect arch around his chin.

The Confederate torpedoes planted at the entrance to Mobile Bay were the first, and were very primitive in their construction—merely a lager beer keg filled with powder and anchored by chains to a big flat piece of iron called a mushroom. Projecting from the swinging top, some four feet under water, were tubes of glass filled with sulphuric acid, and which, being broken, fell into sugar or starch, causing rapid chemical combustion, and finally a mass of fire, thus exploding the powder. They had been planted so long that many leaked, only one out of ten remaining intact, and this fact explains why so many were run over by the Federal fleet without exploding.

During the four months that we were guarding the entrance to Mobile Bay we were not by any means safe from the danger of our contrivances. One hot July morning we officers were up on the flat deck of the ram enjoying the sea breeze, when a floating black object was observed bobbing up and down, and supposed at first that it was a sort of a devilfish with its young, as we had killed one with its calf only a few weeks previously; but the motion was too slow, evidently. A telescope soon revealed the fact that it was a torpedo drifting in with the flood-tide. Here was literally the 'devil to pay!' We could not send a boat's crew after it to tow it out of the way. You could not touch it; you could not guide it. There was no means in our power to divert it from its course.

Finally at the suggestion of Captain David Rainey [Lieutenant David G. Raney] Jr. of the Marines, he brought up his whole guard with loaded muskets, who at once commenced to shoot at the floating keg and sunk it, but not a moment too soon, for it only disappeared under the water about twenty feet from the ram.

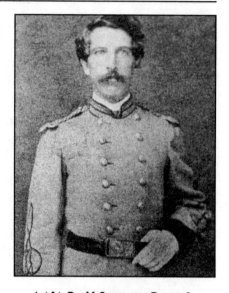

1st Lt. David Greenway Raney, Jr.

Head of the 36 marines that made up the marine guard on the *Tennessee*

Ralph W. Donnelly, *The Confederate States Marine Corps*

There was brought on board the *Tennessee* a complement of marines from the Confederate marine barracks in Mobile. This marine guard consisted of 36 marines, First Lieutenant David G. Raney, Jr., two sergeants, two corporals, one musician, and 30 privates.

As the sketch is confined exclusively to operations inside the shield of the ram *Tennessee*, I have not thought it germane to detail anything in relation to the other three gunboats of the Confederate fleet, which being wooden vessels, were sunk or captured early in the first action.

It may be interesting, which is omitted above, to state the cause of the wound received by Admiral Buchanan. It was by a fragment of iron, either a piece of solid shot, or part of the plating of the ram which fractured the large bone of the leg, comminuting it, and the splintered ends protruding through the muscles and the skin.

The admiral's aides were Lieutenants Carter and Forrest. They tenderly nursed him during the entire four months of his confinement in the hospital at Pensacola, accompanied him to Fort Warren, cared for him while there, and brought him back to Richmond after his exchange. The former is now a prominent citizen of North Carolina; the later until ten years ago lived in Virginia, since which time I have lost sight of him."[2]

Extant is the journal of James C. Palmer, fleet surgeon of the Federal navy at Mobile Bay. In this Dr. Palmer described the battle and the events immediately following:

> We next saw the *Lackawana* battling the *Tennessee*; and then the *Monongahela*, (the sailors called her <u>Monkey</u>—<u>healer</u>) and then the *Hartford* which first rammed, and then as she scraped against the iron sponson [definition: a structure projecting from the side or main deck of a vessel to support a gun] of the *Tennessee*, delivered his shot port broadside into the armour of that vessel, without penetrating it. At last the *Manhattan* delivered her 15-inch shell, which drove deep into the monster, and enabled the *Chickasaw's* 11-inch guns to penetrate. In the mean time, the *Tennessee's* smokestack was shaken down, and her steering apparatus damaged; so after her gallant struggle, she became helpless, and Admiral Buchanan surrendered to the fleet, and sent his sword to Admiral Farragut. (Giraud took it.)
>
> All this occured while I was near the *Richmond* and *Lackawanna*. The *Richmond* had only two men slightly wounded and none killed; aboard the *Lackawanna* however, I saw sights of horror.
>
> The *Richmond* moved to me as I passed back and told me that the Admiral had partly signalled for me to return which I did immediately. When I got near enough to the *Hartford*, the Admiral himself hailed, and directed me to go aboard the captured ram, and look after Admiral Buchanan, who was wounded. It

was difficult, even from a boat to get aboard the *Tennessee* and I had to make a long leap assisted by a strong man's hand. I *scrambled*, literally, through the iron port and threaded my way among piles of confusion to a ladder by which I mounted to where Admiral Buchanan was lying in a place like the triangular top of a Cheops' pyramid. Somebody announced me and he answered (tone polite, but savage) 'I know Dr. Palmer'; but he gave me his hand. I told him I was sorry to see him so badly hurt but that I should be glad to know his wishes. He answered, 'I only wish to be treated kindly as a prisoner of war.' My reply was, 'Admiral Buchanan, you know perfectly well you will be treated kindly.' Then he said, 'I am a Southern man and an enemy and a rebel.' I felt a little offended at his tone but enjoined carefully that he was at that moment, a wounded person, and disabled and that I would engage to have his wishes fulfilled. As to the present disposal of his person, that Admiral Farragut would take him aboard the *Hartford* or send him to any other ship he might prefer. He said he didn't pretend to be Admiral Farragut's friend and had no right to ask favors of him, but that he should be satisfied with any decision that might be come to. As I was taking leave Dr. Conrad, lately an assistant surgeon in our navy, told me he was fleet surgeon and desired to accompany Admiral Buchanan wherever he might go. I promised he should and returned to the *Hartford* and responded to Admiral Farragut circumstantially. This generous man seemed somewhat hurt at Admiral Buchanan's irritated feeling and said he had formerly professed friendship for him. I saw there must be some embarrassment in bringing them together and therefore proposed that I should have a steamer to take the wounded to Pensacola, and another one to send all ordinary invalids from Pensacola to New Orleans so as to leave the hospital at Pensacola clear. This was immediately adopted. Alden was sent to Fort Morgan to get permission for a steamer to pass under flag of truce; and we signalled to the fleet to have all the wounded ready. Then we got all our forces together; and as long as we could see, we were lopping off legs and arms. Dr. Williams, Dr. Lansdale, Dr. Gibson, myself and some assistant surgeons were at it all the afternoon. I think it was about 10 o'clock at night when I left the *Hartford*; then there were 20 dead men lying in a row on the quarter-deck. I took away the body of Captain Drayton's clerk to be buried at Pensacola and three or four heads were thrown overboard, the bodies having been blown to pieces. This would make about 25 killed and I found aboard the *Metacomet*, seventy-one of our own wounded and ten Confederates including Admiral Buchanan. They were all made as comfortable as possible and then kind Jouett fed me and filled me with ale and I blessed God and thought of you and went to sleep.

August 6: Pensacola Navy Yard See how I have marked the date; by that you will know I am safe. About sunrise, we passed in full view of Fort Morgan and put to sea. One of our brave fellows had died during the night leaving seventy wounded aboard. As we neared the *Tennessee*, senior vessel outside, she gave three cheers but Jouett with characteristic delicacy would not mortify our prisoners by returning them. By and by he came to me to ask my advice about putting them on parole and I advised him to let them pledge themselves to Admiral Buchanan. This was done and then he pledged his parole of honor for himself and his people. The following is a copy of the paper handed to me. 'A list of officers and men who have given their parole of honor to

Admiral F. Buchanan not to leave the limits prescribed by those in authority without special permission of Fleet Surgeon J. C. Palmer, U. S. Navy.' Here follows the names of officers and enemy and the whole is signed 'Frank'n Buchanan, Admiral, C. S. N.' Thus everything passed harmoniously but I must tell you in our confidence that <u>Dr. Conrad had prepared Admiral Buchanan's mind to lose his leg and I resisted the sacrifice else it would certainly have been done.</u> It was about 4 in the afternoon when we cleared the *Metacomet* of wounded and happy indeed was I to be back in my own garret again. The pencil marks read, 'God's blessings on you!'

<u>August 7:</u> Admiral Buchanan's leg with Dr. Nathan R. Smith's anterior splint, but not to my satisfaction; there was too much interference and the indications were not observed in a manner to secure a good result.

<u>August 8:</u> Necessary this morning to amputate both the legs of one poor fellow and the ordinary work is quite fatiguing.[3]

Captured on the *Tennessee* were 20 officers and about 170 men. There exists a small Bible that belonged to Dr. Conrad and in the flyleaf of it, Dr. Conrad wrote: "This book was saved from the CS ironclad *Tennessee* after action of August 5th, 1864."

The following memorandum was written by Admiral Buchanan after he had recuperated and was heading off to the Northern prison, Fort Lafayette. This small note was given to Dr. Conrad.

<u>Concerning</u> the statements of the Northern press as to the number of vessels engaged, several of these statements say Admiral Buchanan's fleet consisted of three ironclads, three cotton clads and other vessels. None of the fleet chased the *Tennessee*. They

passed her, we fighting them as they passed and when they anchored in the bay the *Tennessee* followed them alone and renewed the action. The crew was not demoralized as one account stated. The men stood tall and by to their guns and brought them to the last moment as cheerfuly as they commenced the action. They were all from the army and had been in many hard fought battles and were therefore not be alarmed by the smell of gun powder or the sight of dead men. No officers or men ever went into a fight with better spirits. The enemy had 14 steamers and four monitors in the fight carrying 199 heavy guns and a number of brass howitzers in the top and on other parts of the ships and 3,000 men. The little Mobile Squadron had 22 guns and 470 men. The enemy lost nearly 300 in killed and wounded exclusive of the 120 lost in the *Tecumseh* blown up by a torpedo. The Mobile Squadron 10 killed and 19 wounded. Admiral Buchanan's sword was delivered to Captain Giraud, [Acting Volunteer Lieutenant Pierre Giraud] the officer who was sent on board to take charge of the *Tennessee* after the surrender and was not delivered to any officer on board the *Hartford* by Captain Johnston as Admiral Farragut says in his report. Captain Giraud asked for the sword by direction of Admiral Farragut and it was delivered to him by one of Admiral Buchanan's aides.

Memorandum
for
Dr. Conrad
_____

Ad. Buchanan to
<u>Cert.</u> Surg. D. B. Conrad
Pensacola Hospital
October 1864

[Dr. Conrad wrote]

> Given me on my being sent
> thru the lines to Mobile
> He was sent to prison
> Fort Lafayette[4]

Admiral Buchanan wrote from the hospital at Pensacola on August 26, "...Fleet-Surgeon D. B. Conrad, to whom I am much indebted for his skill, promptness and attention to the wounded. By permission of Admiral Farragut he accompanied the wounded of the *Tennessee* and *Selma* to this hospital, and is assisted by Assistant-Surgeons Booth and Bowles of the *Selma* and *Tennessee*, all under the charge of Fleet-Surgeon Palmer, of the United States Navy, from whom we have received all the attention and consideration we could desire or expect."[5] Conrad was given the above note by Admiral Buchanan before Conrad was sent by flag of truce back to Mobile in October. Buchanan was carried at the end of November to Fort Lafayette and imprisoned."

Dr. Conrad received the following letter from Admiral Buchanan's wife:

> Home
>
> Sept 21st, '64.
>
> Your very welcome letter, my dear doctor reached me yesterday. I am partly cheered by and reading your account of your patient, to you & Doctor P., & kind attention & skill (as far as human means goes). I am sure his leg, as well as life, has been saved. I trust he will continue to do well—but I can not help feeling very anxious as the time draws near for removing the bandage, to learn if the bone has united properly and when he can stand & walk on it. If it does not, what will be the result? Please let me hear as soon as this is ascertained.
>
> I am much disappointed and disturbed that I am not permitted to be his nurse. I know I could have saved you much trouble. I dread much the time, when you must be removed to those Northern Bastiles and

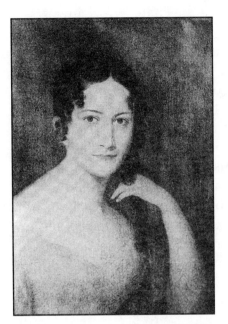

Mrs. Anne Catherine Lloyd Buchanan

She wrote a letter thanking Dr. Conrad for all he had done for her husband after he was wounded at Mobile Bay.

Charles Lee Lewis,
Admiral Franklin Buchanan

Dr. Richard Curd Bowles

He served as assistant surgeon under Dr. Conrad on the *Tennessee*.
Carte-de-visite of Richard Bowles, Jr.

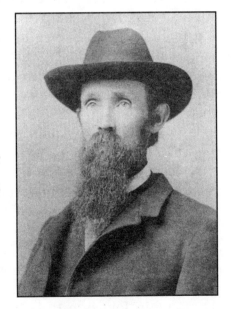

am selfish enough to hope you are to be one of the party and am willing to make the change [for] any of you all.

Great as the risk be—as false as it might be—a little risk for body & mind is sometimes useful, you know. Maybe you will call on me as your Mother, if I can in any way contribute to your comfort in fitting up your clothes, warmest & suitable for a cold climate. So far as the rules of prison life permits and as I hope to do for my husband. I see your cousins very often. They are our most intimate & kindest friends. I hope you get Louisa's letter. She was as kind as to send it to me & it was the first true account I had of his situation.

Most Respectfully
& Truly Yours,
N. Buchanan[6]

Serving on the *Tennessee* with Conrad, as his assistant surgeon was Dr. Richard Curd Bowles of Hanover County, Virginia. Dr. Bowles recounted the wounding of Admiral Buchanan and the final moments of the Battle of Mobile Bay from his perspective within the *Tennessee*. He also remembers the Captain's name as Johnson not Johnston; herein corrected.

A messenger comes to inform us that the Admiral is wounded; he is brought on the berth deck and placed on a mattress. We find he has a fracture of the leg. He had a similar wound in the *Merrimac* fight. In a short time, a messenger comes from Captain Johnston, saying the ship is disabled, and he thinks we had better surrender. The old Admiral rouses up, sparks seem to flash from his eyes, he brings his clinched fist down on the deck, 'Go back and tell Captain Johnston to fight the ship to the very last man.' Soon the captain came himself, and told the Admiral the ship would be sunk in five minutes if he did not surrender. He replied sadly, 'I leave the whole matter to you, Captain Johnston.' The Captain then tied his white handkerchief to the ramrod of a musket, and pushed it up through the hatchway. Unfortunately the noise was so great that the order to cease firing had not been understood, and one of our guns fired after the white flag had been raised.

The Federal officer who came aboard to receive the surrender of the ship demanded why this had been done, and talked of taking summary vengeance on us, but Captain Johnston's explanation seemed to satisfy him.

Mr. Forrest of Virginia, master's mate, learning that the ship was about to surrender, ran down and begged the Admiral to give him his sword. He did not want Farragut to have it. He made no reply, but Mr. Forrest unbuckled the sword and threw it out of the port hole...As soon as Farragut heard that the Admiral was wounded he sent his fleet surgeon aboard, offering assistance. This was very kind of him. Indeed, they accorded us generous treatment as men worthy of their steel and soon the Blue and the Gray were fraternizing in the most friendly manner...

Admiral Buchanan united with Farragut in a petition to General Page at Fort Morgan to allow a ship to pass out with Federal and Confederate wounded to Pensacola, Florida, where they could be made more comfortable. To this he assented. All the wounded having been tranferred to the U. S. steamer *Metacomet* on the morning of the 6th of August, we sailed for Pensacola with a full cargo of mutilated and suffering humanity."[7]

Admiral Farragut, on his flagship *Hartford*, lamented on August 22, 1864, that, "The Rebels, I understand refuse to exchange our Navy officers except for [their] Navy officers..."

He still had the three surgeons captured at the Battle of Mobile Bay, "...Fleet Surgeon Conrad, Assistant Surgeons R. C. Bowles and E. G. Booth."[8]

Farragut from the *Hartford* on September 12, while still at Mobile Bay, wrote to his superiors explaining his treatment of Dr. Conrad and Admiral Buchanan.

> Flagship *Hartford*
> Mobile Bay, Sept. 12, 1864
>
> Commodore:
>
> ...My understanding was that Surgeon Conrad should be allowed to attend the wounds of Admiral Buchanan so long as his services were needed for that purpose and should then be permitted to return on parole to this place, and thence to Mobile, upon the ground that a surgeon's mission was one of mercy, and because similar acts of courtesy have been extended to our medical officers by the enemy. I do not admit, however, that the fleet surgeon is responsible for anything more than the medical care and condition of the prisoners, as they are well enough to be moved he should report the same to you, in order that you may dispose of them as may have been directed.
>
> I did not fail to call Lieutenant-Commander Jouett to account for taking those medical officers on board at the request of the fleet surgeon without orders from you. I do not permit any one to be taken on board a vessel within my reach without written orders to the commanding officer. The permission granted Surgeon Conrad was a courtesy to Admiral Buchanan and to insure him against the chance of mismanagement of his case, then understood to be critical.
>
> Very respectfully,
> D. G. Farragut
> Rear-Admiral[9]

Dr. Richard Curd Bowles

Richard Curd Bowles, the son of Abraham Perkins Bowles and Betsy Richardson Bowles, was born in Hanover County on May 6, 1837. He studied medicine at the University of Maryland and graduated in 1860.

Early in the Civil War, Dr. Bowles enlisted as a private in Company D of the 44th Virginia Infantry. In May of 1862, however, Dr. Bowles transferred to the Confederate navy where he could put his medical skills to use. For a brief period, he served as a staff surgeon in one of the many hospitals that sprung up around Richmond during the war.

On Christmas Day, 1863, Dr. Bowles was ordered to report to Mobile Bay to serve as assistant surgeon on the ironclad *Tennessee*. Seven months later, Dr. Bowles found himself in the middle of one of the largest naval battles of the Civil War...After the battle and his capture by Federal forces, Dr. Bowles was ordered to join the naval forces along the James River. He was captured once again during the evacuation of Richmond, but escaped and walked home.

After the war, Dr. Bowles embarked upon the life of a country doctor...he died on June 8, 1923, having practiced medicine in Goochland for almost fifty years...[10]

On November 1, 1864, the surgeon in charge, W.A.W. Spotswood, wrote to the Honorable S. R. Mallory, secretary of the navy, in Richmond and reported Fleet Surgeon Conrad was the only surgeon in the fleet off Mobile.[11]

After Buchanan surrendered, the command of the remaining naval squadron near Mobile was under Flag Officer Ebenezer Farrand.

Farrand took the remainder of his small force up the Alabama River and into the Tombigbee. They went up as far as Nanna Hubba Bluffs, and there they awaited developments. Commodore Henry K. Thatcher, who had replaced Farragut in command of the West Gulf Blockading Squadron, sent up a couple monitors to watch the Confederate vessels but made no attempt to attack them. Finally, on May 8, nearly a month after Appomattox, Farrand surrendered to the Union naval officer.[12]

Dr. Daniel B. Conrad was still with the Mobile squadron when it was surrendered and he was paroled at Nanna Hubba, Alabama, on May 10, 1865.

Chapter Seven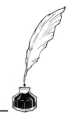

The Years after the War

What Dr. Conrad did the few years immediately after the Civil War is unclear. Conrad probably returned to his family home in Winchester where he practiced medicine for about five years. His interests soon turned to the care of the mentally ill. He called on one of his staunchest friends and his ex-patient, Franklin Buchanan, for a letter of recommendation to submit to his prospective employer. Former Confederate Admiral Franklin Buchanan wrote from Mobile, Alabama, on February 22, 1870, a letter to the board of directors, Eastern Insane Asylum, Williamsburg, Virginia, recommending Dr. Conrad for the position of superintendent of that institution.[1] Evidently, Dr. Conrad did not get that job, but did take the superintendency at the newly formed hospital in Richmond for the insane black population of Virginia.

It was urged as early as 1845, by many progressive physicians including Dr. Francis T. Stribling, the superintendent of the Western Insane Asylum, at Staunton, that the state of Virginia establish an insane asylum for its black inhabitants. After the Civil War, with the encouragement of Dr. Hunter McGuire, Major General Edward Richard Sprigg Canby, the military governor of Virginia, decreed that blacks in need of psychiatric treatment be taken to an old Confederate hospital, Howard's Grove Freedman's Hospital.[2] This hospital was established on a popular Richmond recreation area which had been turned by the authorities into a drill and bivouac site. This area was converted into a Confederate hospital and after constructing 62 buildings, the hospital opened for patients in June of 1862. It had an initial capacity of 659 patients but the hospital was quickly expanded to 1,800 beds.[3] It was located on the northeastern outskirts of Richmond on the Mechanicsville Turnpike near the area of what is now 25th and T Streets.

On June 7, 1870, the Central Lunatic Asylum was incorporated by the following law, "Be it enacted by the general assembly, That a lunatic asylum is hereby established, to be located temporarily at Howard's Grove, near the city of Richmond, which shall be for the reception and treatment of colored persons of unsound mind..." Dr. Daniel Burr Conrad was selected as the first superintendent of this new temporary hospital and assumed charge on July 1, 1870. The old Confederate hospital consisting of a couple wooden, one-story buildings were whitewashed inside and outside. Dr. Conrad immediately built, "sheds, four in number, in which the meals were served." Also built were "...a stable and cow-house, coal-house and

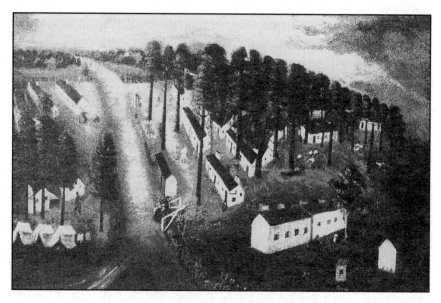

Howard's Grove Freedman's Hospital

The hospital was established for the care of Virginia's black mentally ill patients. It was an old Confederate hospital.

Chicago Historical Society

piggery, with sheds for laundry and kitchen." Conrad also built another story on the buildings thereby doubling the hospital's inmate capacity. Heat was supplied by large coal-burning stoves and light by kerosene lamps and tallow candles. The Howard's Grove Hospital was leased from the owner of the land on which it was located. The lease was unclear as to the ownership of any new buildings or improvements to the existing buildings when the lease ran out. Therefore, Dr. Conrad recommended a committee be appointed "to examine into and report immediately for their future action regarding the selection of a site and the erection of a permanent asylum for the colored insane of the state."[4]

On November 14, 1871, Dr. Conrad married Susan Lymon Davis of Newtown, at Stephens City, in Frederick County, Virginia. Susan was the daughter of Dr. William Augustus Davis. They were married by the Reverend W. C. Meredith at "Sunny Side."

Dr. Davis had moved to Winchester from Massachusetts in 1856. Dr. Davis had been in the Massachusetts militia before the war and his militia coat and pants are now in the Warren Rifles Confederate Museum in Front Royal, Virginia. Susan Davis had been a young girl of 19 or 20 years of age when General Philip Sheridan's men raided her parents' farm at Sunnyside and stole their only milk cow. Fiesty young Susan mounted the family mule, stormed into the camp of General Philip Sheridan, and demanded the return of the cow, which was promptly returned. The following is another anecdotal

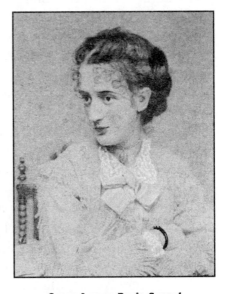

Susan Lymon Davis Conrad

A tinted likeness of the wife of Dr. Daniel B. Conrad

Carte-de-visite in Author's Collection

story passed down through the family. It took place at the time that Susan's brother and father were away serving in the Confederate army. A Yankee officer became an admirer of the family and posted a 24-hour guard at the house to prevent property damage by rampaging Yankee soldiers.

For most of the war, Dr. Davis served in the Confederate army in the Valley of Virginia and at Chimborazo Hospital in Richmond. The authorities began Chimborazo General Hospital after the start of the Civil War and its first patients were admitted on October 17, 1861. The normal occupancy of the hospital was about three thousand patients. It had a medical staff of about 45 and handled about 17,000 wounded cases during its existence.[5] Dr. Davis was at one time the Chief surgeon for Division #4.[6] In July 1862, Division #4 had a patient capacity of three hundred but at that time, only 222 beds were occupied.[7] Dr. Davis was a member of the "Board of Consulting Surgeons for Chimborazo." He was a member of the Reserve Surgical Corps based in Richmond, but was temporarily detached in July 1864, and sent back to the Shenandoah Valley to establish a hospital if needed to care for any "sudden outbursts of wounded."[8]

Dr. Davis and Dr. Conrad knew each other well enough to help form a professional organization while serving together in Richmond. Dr. Conrad had served with Dr. Davis as an officer in an organization called The Army and Navy Surgeons of the Confederate States that they helped form in Richmond in 1864. Later at Danville, near the end of the war, Dr. Davis would be severely wounded by an explosion while trying to save medical supplies.

On November 15, 1873, after three years' service, Dr. Conrad retired from the hospital at Howard's Grove because of ill health. The board of directors, under which Conrad served, passed the following resolution: "That this board accepts, with a sincere regret, the resignation of Dr. D. B. Conrad, the present superintendent of this institution, and that it be recorded as the sense of this board that he has discharged the difficult duties devolved upon him with skill and fidelity."[9]

This temporary asylum was occupied until a permanent site was selected on land bought by the city of Petersburg and donated to the state in 1882. In 1885, Central State Hospital, about a mile west of Petersburg, opened its doors for Negroes in need of psychiatric treatment. Hanging in the hall of the main Administration Building of Central State Hospital in Petersburg [in 1995] is an oil portrait of Dr. Conrad.

Dr. Conrad was involved in the controversy of the procurement of cadavers from the insane asylum where he was superintendent. The bodies were used for dissection by the medical students in Richmond.

> ...in 1880, there was considerable excitement in Richmond, accompanied by newspaper publicity concerning the activities of the resurrectionists in Oakwood Cemetery. As early as 1878, Surgeon Conrad, of the colored insane asylum, had complained to Keeper W. L. Smith of Oakwood that the body of a patient of his had been taken from the cemetery and had later been identified by a student in the dissecting room of the Medical College of Virginia.[10]

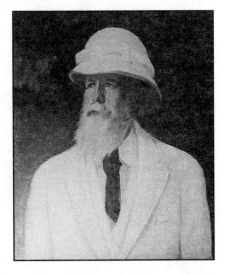

Painting of Dr. Daniel Burr Conrad

This oil painting hangs in the hall of the modern administrative office at the Central State Mental Hospital in Petersburg, Virginia.

Author's Photograph

Later because of his previous experience, Dr. Conrad was selected as the superintendent of the Western Lunatic Asylum, now known as Western State Hospital, Staunton, Virginia, from April 1, 1886, through April 21, 1889.[11]

Dr. and Mrs. Conrad had her father as a guest in their home in the 1870s and 1880s

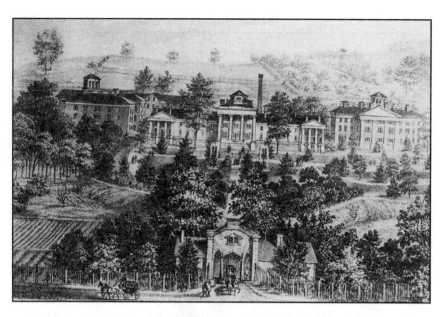

Western State Hospital

Dr. Conrad came out of retirement to take the superintendency of this hospital located in Staunton, Virginia.

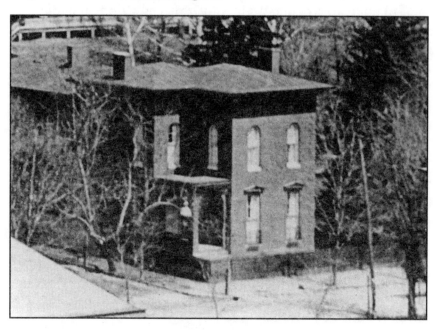

House of Dr. Daniel Burr Conrad

Located on West Boscawen Street, in Winchester, Virginia, about 1900 and this caused friction between Conrad and his father-in-law. They lived in a large brick home on the northeast corner of Boscawen Street and Stewart Street at 230 West Boscawen Street.

It was said the two doctors seldom spoke to each other during this time. In any event, Dr. Conrad left without his wife and moved to 916 Tracy Street, Kansas City, Missouri, from 1891 through 1898. His application for a Missouri license on January 26, 1891, stated he would practice allopathic medicine and at the present age of 60, he had practiced medicine 39 years.[12]

Allopathic medicine was the philosophy of medicine that believed that the best method of treating disease was by the use of agents producing effects or symptoms exactly opposite to those of the disease being treated, whereas homeopathic medicine was treating with agents that produce the same effects as the disease being treated. Dr. Conrad was in need of an affidavit certifying that he had received a doctor of medicine degree from the University of Pennsylvania. On January 22, 1891, this institution furnished him such an affidavit, "It being understood that the diploma of said Daniel B. Conrad has been lost."

This was used by Daniel Conrad, who resided in Jackson County, to obtain from the Missouri State Board of Health a license to practice medicine. It was issued on the third day of February 1891, in St. Louis.[13]

Conrad wrote possibly a dozen interesting articles for the local newspaper, the *Winchester Times*. Among them was one published in June 1890, titled, "Thomas Lord Fairfax, Lord Proprietor of the Northern Neck of Virginia 1745 and Founder of the City of Winchester." Another, by Conrad while in Kansas, was printed in the paper in June 1893, titled, "Selim, the Algerine, A Waif of Colonial Virginia." On Wednesday, July 5, 1893, he wrote in the *Winchester Times*, "Peter Muldenburg," telling the life of this Revolutionary War hero. Other articles published by Dr. Conrad are the five or six previously mentioned, i.e., "Torpedo Attack, by Lieutenant Glassell," "First

Manassas," "Mobile Bay," and "The *Underwriter.*" One appeared in the "Patriotic Youths Department" section of the January 1895 *Blue and Gray* magazine, titled "General Daniel Morgan, The 'Thunderbolt of the Revolution.'" It told the story of the patriot from the Valley of Virginia whose escapades were "known to every school child" at that time.

Conrad wrote a very interesting montage of about six short vignettes in a monthly periodical called *The United Service,* a monthly review of military and naval affairs. These stories were included in 11 pages of the October 1892 issue titled "Some Yarns Spun by an Officer of the Old Navy." One yarn told the amusing story of "Jamaica Tom" a very large man-eating shark that loved to roam the waters of Kingston, Jamaica. "Jamaica Tom" prevented the common practice of sailors jumping ship at night and going ashore for some nocturnal bar hopping. This massive old shark defied all attempts to kill it. Harpoons would glance off, bullets never found their mark, and baited hooks would bend. Some sailors noticed that "Tom" would almost jump up out of the water to get a large slab of pork skin. The cook decided to have the ship's tailor make a large purse or envelope-shaped container and into this container they put a red-hot six-pound cannonball. They lowered this over the side of the ship and "Tom" swallowed it in one gulp. "Tom" suffering from a severe stomachache, dove down and returned to the surface several times for the next hour or so and finally went belly up. All the sailors felt free thereafter to dive overboard and to swim to and from shore each night.[14]

Some time in 1898, Dr. Daniel Conrad returned home. Dr. Conrad died of longstanding Bright's disease (kidney disease or glomerulonephritis) at 8:30 o'clock in the morning of September 20, 1898, at his residence on West Water (now Boscawen) Street, Winchester.[15]

Mrs. Susan D. Conrad lived a long and fruitful life after her husband died. Besides his wife, Dr. Conrad was survived by three sons and three daughters. Susan Conrad was active in many civic and philanthropic endeavors for three decades after her husband died.

Dr. Conrad's grave is marked by a large towering cross headstone shared with his wife at the venerable Mount Hebron Cemetery in Winchester.

Dr. Daniel Burr Conrad was one of the three or four principal medical officers of the Civil War. Though Conrad never received the recognition that was due him, he was one of the few truly heroic fighting medical officers of the Confederacy.

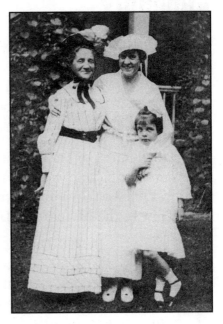

Susan Lymon Davis

This photograph of the wife of Dr. Daniel B. Conrad with her daughter, Eleanor Barnard Conrad Carson, and her granddaughter, Susan Davis Carson Hedrick, was taken in 1915, outside the Conrad home in Winchester, Virginia.

Author's Collection

Appendix

Genealogy and Miscellaneous Information

Groupings of information or clippings will be separated by asterisks.

Daniel Burr Conrad was a member of the Kent Street Presbyterian Church and was buried in the beautiful old Mount Hebron Cemetery in Winchester, Virginia.

Below is the obituary of Dr. Conrad:

DEATH OF DR. D. B. CONRAD
A Former Surgeon in the Navy
Also Served on the Staff of Admiral Buchanan.

Dr. Daniel Burr Conrad, one of the most prominent citizens of this place, died on last Tuesday morning at 8:30 o'clock at his residence on West Water Street, from Bright's disease, after being sick for about nine months. Dr. Conrad, besides being a very prominent physician, was also a writer of considerable note, he having contributed articles to the *Army and Navy Magazine*, the *Blue and the Gray* and various New York papers.

Dr. Conrad was a son of the late Robt. Y. Conrad. He was born in this city in 1831. He received his education at the Winchester Academy, from which school he graduated, and afterward took the academic course at the University of Virginia. He then began the study of medicine at the Winchester Medical College, taking the degree of M. D., and afterward took a post-graduate course at the Jefferson Medical College, Philadelphia. At the age of 25 he was appointed a surgeon in the United States Navy and served on the *Congress* and *Brooklyn.* He has cruised all over the world and was surgeon on the boat that took the first Japanese delegation that ever visited this country back to Japan. When he returned to this country the Civil War had broken out, and he resigned his commission.

Dr. Conrad was appointed a surgeon in the Second Virginia Regiment, Confederate army, which place he held for about five months and was appointed surgeon in the Confederate navy and placed on Admiral Buchanan's staff. He was in all the large naval battles in the Civil War, and when at the battle of Mobile Bay, January, 1865, Admiral Buchanan had his leg shattered, Dr. Conrad amputated it. He was also at the capture and burning of the U. S. Gunboat *Underwriter* at Newbern Bay in January, 1864.

After the war he was appointed superintendent of the lunatic asylum now located at Petersburg, but then located at Richmond. After filling this position for a number of years he resigned on account of ill health. He was also Superintendent, of the Western State Hospital at Staunton, for three years, when he resigned.

In 1871 he married Miss Susie Davis, daughter of the late Dr. Wm. A. Davis. Six children, Mrs. Henry Little of Norfolk; Misses Bessie and Eleanor and Messrs. Robert Y., Daniel B. Jr., and William Davis Conrad, besides his wife surived him. He also leaves three brothers, Maj. Holmes, Frank E. and Chas. Conrad of Tennessee, and two sisters, Miss Kate Conrad and Mrs. Fauntleroy of Staunton. Dr. Conrad was a member of the Kent Street Presbyterian Church.

The funeral of the late Dr. Daniel B. Conrad took place from his late residence on Water Street at 4 o'clock on Thursday afternoon. Rev. Dr. James R. Graham, assisted by Rev. Nelson P. Dame, conducted the services.[1]

Daniel Conrad was survived by his wife, Susan L. Conrad, and by three sons:

Daniel Burr Conrad, Jr.—of Winchester.

William Davis Conrad—lawyer, of New York City.

Robert Y. Conrad—

and three daughters:

Mrs. Henry H. Little (Annie Middleton Conrad)—of Norfolk. She was the eldest of Dr. Conrad's daughters. Had a daughter Susan Conrad Little, who had a daughter Mary McGeorge Little Bundy, who had a daughter Anne Bundy Lewis of Petersburg.

Mrs. Adam Clarke Carson, ("Miss Eleanor" Barnard Conrad)—of Riverton, Virginia. Adam Clarke (age 39) was born in Ulster, Ireland, and was a resident of Manila, Philippine Islands, where he was assistant superintendent of colonial affairs. He married Eleanor Conrad (age 25) on May 12, 1908, and they made their home at "Dellbrook." They had a daughter Susan who married John S. Hedrick and they had a daughter, Miss Caroline Carson. Both Adam Clarke Carson, and his wife, Eleanor Conrad Carson, are buried in Front Royal in Prospect Hill Cemetery. Adam Clarke Carson was buried in 1941 and Eleanor Conrad Carson in 1950.

Miss Elizabeth "Bessie" Whiting Conrad—of Winchester.

* * * * * * * * *

Daniel B. Conrad's siblings were:

(a) Powell Conrad—born in 1833—lawyer—served as engineer for Ashby's Cavalry—Died in service on May 21, 1862, of typhoid fever. Buried in the graveyard of the University of Virginia near Charlottesville, Virginia.

(b) Catherine "Kate" B. Conrad—born April 2, 1836, lived in Staunton; engaged to Captain Richard Ashby, brother of Confederate General Turner Ashby.

(c) Robert Y. Conrad—born in 1836—graduate of the University of Virginia; died November 14, 1858.

(d) Holmes Conrad—born 1840—E. Holmes Bond, wrote from Winchester, Virginia, in March 1908 that Holmes had "...enlisted in Newtown Cavalry (a Frederick county company), First Virginia Regiment of Cavalry (J. E. B. Stuart's old regiment); became adjutant of the Eleventh Virginia Cavalry, commissioned major and served on the staff of General Thomas L. Rosser; practiced law in Winchester until 1893; member of the Legislature, Assistant Attorney General and Solicitor General under President Cleveland, and was a resident of Winchester, but maintained his law office in Washington, D. C."—married in Maryland, to Georgia Bryan Forman, daughter of Thomas Bryan Forman, of Savannah, Georgia.

(e) Sally Harrison Conrad—born July 2, 1842—engaged to Henry Kyd Douglas, but she married Dr. Archibald Magill Fauntleroy in Winchester on April 26, 1866. They moved to Staunton, Augusta County, Virginia, where Dr. Fauntleroy was a practicing physician for 15 years. Afterwards he became superintendent of the Western State Lunatic Asylum in Staunton.

(f) Charles Frederick Conrad—born in 1844—served as a member of Chew's Battery of Horse Artillery—engineer in the Army of Tennessee—married May Louisa Grant, of Savannah, Georgia. After the war he became a civil engineer, and in March 1908, was residing at Staunton.

(g) Francis Edward "Frank" Conrad—born in 1846—served as a member of Chew's Battery, was a lawyer and civil engineer—married Daisy Harrison of Leesburg, Virginia.

(h) Cuthbert Powell Conrad—born 1848—teacher—married Miss Sara Harris of Kansas City; died July 1891.[2]

Daniel Burr Conrad's father, Robert Young Conrad, lived and died in the town where he was born, occupying the same house during a life of 69 years and five months. He married

Elizabeth Whiting Powell on December 10, 1829. He died on Wednesday, May 5, 1875, at half past three in the evening. He was buried by his wife, Elizabeth Whiting Conrad, who was born August 10. She died in Winchester, July 12, 1872.[3]

* * * * * * * * * *

Dr. Conrad's wife lived a full and long life after the death of her husband. She died on Thursday, September 15, 1927. Her obituary in the *Winchester Evening Star* the next day, follows:

MRS. D. B. CONRAD PASSES AWAY AFTER
A BRIEF ILLNESS

End Comes Quietly and Peacefully to One Long Prominent In Church, Social and Literary Circles; Funeral Services Saturday Afternoon; Came of a Distinguished Massachusetts Family, Locating Here Just Before Outbreak of Civil War.

Mrs. Daniel Burr Conrad, widow of Dr. Conrad, died last night at her home here on Boscawen Street, in the eighty-third year of her age. Surrounded by her children and and grandchildren, mentally conscious and clear almost to the last, she slept peacefully into the new life which she believed awaited her.

Mrs. Conrad was ill only ten days, and really died from the accumulating weaknesses of old age. Her mind remained vigorous and young, while her body became weak and old; indeed, her interests in men and things inspired and informed her reading and conversation until a little more than a week ago.

Mrs. Conrad is survived by two sons, W. Davis Conrad, a New York Lawyer, and Daniel Burr Conrad, of Winchester, and by three daughters, Mrs. Henry H. Little, of Norfolk, Va., Mrs. A. C. Carson, of Riverton, Va., and Miss Elizabeth Whiting Conrad, of Winchester.

The funeral services will be held at Christ Episcopal Church, of which Mrs. Conrad was long a member, at 4 o'clock tomorrow afternoon. Rev. Robert B. Nelson officiating. Following an old custom in the Conrad family, reminiscent of the older Virginia, the active pallbearers will be colored men. These men, who held a high regard for Mrs. Conrad, are: Charles Lampkins, Andrew Cook, John Morris, Charles Williams, Nathaniel Cook, Richard Washington, Edward Jefferson and Joe Willis.

The honorary pallbearers will be Dr. B. B. Dutton, R. Gray Williams, Robert M. Ward, Dr. E. C. Stuart, Charles L. Bowly, Edmund P. Hunter, Dr. Julian F. Ward, Harry F. Byrd, T. W. Harrison, Gray Beverley, Joseph DuPuy, Thomas B. Byrd, William E. Carson, Phillip Williams, Dr. Hunter H. McGuire, Nelson Page, Samuel Authur, Stuart Hunter, H. N. Stephenson, James B. Russell, H. D. Fuller, T. Russell Cather, H. B. McCormac, H. K. Russell, Frank Tilford, Alexander Barrie, Lewis F. Cooper, Henry H. Little, William Beverley, Roland Ryan, E. W. Cather, A. T. Jones, and W. A. Baker.

It was the strange fate of Mrs. Conrad's father and brother to come from New England to Virginia and fight for their adopted state against their native section. Mrs. Conrad's father was Dr. William A. Davis. A man of culture, he graduated in 1837 from Harvard and took his medical degree at the Boston Medical School in 1840. He was, indeed, a Phi Beta Kappa, receiving this recognition at Harvard of his mental attainments.

Dr. Davis practiced his profession a few years in Dorchester and Springfield, Mass., and then determined, only a few years before the outbreak of the Civil War, to move to Virginia. He came to Winchester, bringing with him the little girl, then about twelve, who was to marry Dr. Daniel Burr Conrad, and a son, Charles Barnard Davis, who was to give his life for his adopted state. For a time they lived at the home now owned by Dr. P. W. Boyd, near the house where Mrs. Conrad died before moving to "Sunnyside," the home at Stephens City purchased by Dr. Davis.

It was in this country home, afterwards owned by Dudley Miller, that Mrs. Conrad and her mother suffered the strain and sorrow of war. Doctor Davis had been led by his convictions, although a New England man, to become a surgeon in the Confederate Army, and his son, at 18, had become a private in Company F, Seventh Virginia Cavalry. With father and son in the army, the mother and daughter faced alone the trials of life in a country often occupied by the enemy. Dr. Davis carried to his death the wounds he suffered at Danville, when he was in an explosion trying to save medical stores, while his son was killed in battle at Road's Hill [sic Rudes Hill], near New Market, only a few weeks before the surrender at Appomattox.

These experiences, these sufferings, these intimate relations with Virginia's part in the Civil War emphasized the undiminished loyalty Mrs. Conrad always retained for the weight and honesty of the convictions felt by the Virginians of that day and the nobility and fineness of their conduct.

Mrs. Conrad's husband was Dr. Daniel Burr Conrad, a son of Robert Y. Conrad, the distinguished Virginia lawyer, and a brother of Major Holmes Conrad, a lawyer of national distinction. They were married some years after the Civil War.

Doctor Conrad attended the University of Virginia, graduated in medicine at the Philadelphia

School of the University of Pennsylvania in 1852, and entered the United States Navy as an assistant surgeon. In 1861 he promptly resigned to return to defend his native state.

In the Confederate Navy he served with rare distinction. When he retired from active service he came to Winchester to live with his family in the home in which Mrs. Conrad died yesterday, and where she had lived nearly fifty years.

Mrs. Conrad held a peculiar place of dignity and influence in this community. For her everyone had respect and her example of elevated life, high ideals and kindly consideration for the rights and feelings of all sort and conditions of men won the admiration of everyone. The best blood of Masssachusetts and Virginia mingled in her veins and gave to her womanhood qualities of pride without arrogance and graciousness without familiarity.

Mrs. Conrad's interests were as varied as an intelligent study of Virginia genealogy and the practical working of a garden. Her mind was alert and her mental curiosity led her reading over a wide field. She wrote from time to time and wrote well.

In August, 1910, Mrs. Conrad made the long trip to the Philippines to visit her daughter, the wife of Judge Adam C. Carson, then a member of the Supreme Court of the islands. She remained active until a few weeks before her death.

Mrs. Conrad had a deep religious faith. She was a Christian without pretense, who lived the principles of this profession. From her life radiated the light of a good example, and now that this light has gone out, the afterflow will linger in the hearts of her friends, a gentle reminder of the gracious personality that was the precious possession of this community for more than a half century.[4]

This obituary was written by her son, W. Burr Conrad, editor of the *Winchester Star*.

* * * * * * * * * *

Extant in the author's collection is a pass or safeguard issued in 1862, to Dr. Conrad's future mother-in-law by the Federal forces occupying Winchester at that time:

Provost Marshal Office
Winchester, Va. April 1862

A safeguard is hereby granted to Mrs. Wm. A. Davis for two passes. All officers and soldiers belonging to the army of the United States are therefore commmanded to respect this safeguard and to afford if necessary protection to the person family and aforementioned property as the case may be. Given at Provost Marshal's office this 22nd of April 1862 in the town of Winchester.

J. H. Lockwoood, Provost Marshal
Maj. 7th Regt. Va. Vol. U.S.A.

By Command of the Marshal
Lieutenant Lewis W. Garett
Provost Lieutenant 11th Regt. P.V.[5]

Notes

CHAPTER ONE

1. Virginia Library, Special Collections Department, Alderman Library, Charlottesville, Virginia.
2. Wyndham B. Blanton, M.D., *Medicine in Virginia in the Nineteenth Century* (Richmond, Va.: Garrett & Massie, Incorporated, 1933), p. 18.
3. Ibid., p. 10.
4. Ibid.
5. Ibid., p. 19.
6. Ibid., p. 10.
7. Author's collection.
8. Ibid.
9. Donald G. Shomette, *Shipwrecks of the Civil War* (Washington, D.C.: Donic Ltd., 1973), pp. 43, 44.
10. Two-volume diary of Dr. Daniel Burr Conrad, Library of Congress, Washington, D.C. Hereafter cited as Conrad Diary.
11. Ibid.
12. Virginia Historical Society.
13. Author's collection.
14. Ibid.
15. Private collection.
16. Ibid.
17. Ibid.
18. Ibid.
19. Ibid.
20. Ibid.
21. Ibid.

CHAPTER TWO

1. Virginia Historical Society.
2. Private collection.
3. Ibid.
4. Conrad Diary.
5. Ibid.
6. National Archives.
7. "Governor's Letters," Virginia State Library Archives, Richmond, Virginia.

CHAPTER THREE

1. Lee A. Wallace, Jr., *A Guide to Virginia Military Organizations, 1861–1865* (Lynchburg, Va.: H. E. Howard, Incorporated, 1986), p. 176.
2. Document in possession of the author.
3. Wallace, p. 176.
4. Daniel Burr Conrad, *Southern Historical Society Papers*, "The History of the First Battle of Manassas and the Organization of the Stonewall Brigade," vol. 19, pp. 82–92. Hereafter cited as *SHSP*.
5. Peter W. Houck, *Confederate Surgeon, The Personal Recollections of E. A. Craighill* (Lynchburg, Va.: H. E. Howard, Inc., 1989), pp. 21, 22.
6. Military Records obtained from the National Archives.
7. Ibid.
8. Document in possession of the author.
9. John W. Schildt, *Hunter Holmes McGuire, Doctor in Gray* (Chewsville, Md.: 1986), p. 26.
10. Private collection.
11. Document in possession of the author.
12. Ibid.
13. Donald G. Shomette, *Shipwrecks of the Civil War* (Washington, D.C.: Donic Ltd., 1973), pp. 327–29.
14. Naval Historical Center.
15. Document in possession of the author.
16. Donald G. Shomette, *Shipwrecks of the Civil War* (Washington, D.C.: Donic Lt. 1973), pp. 294, 295.
17. Ibid., p. 129.
18. Document in possession of the author.
19. *SHSP*, vol. 30, p. 232.
20. Document in possession of the author.
21. Virginia Historical Society.
22. Naval Historical Center.
23. Ibid.
24. Virginia Historical Society.
25. Ibid.
26. Document in possession of the author.
27. Blanton, p. 100.
28. Virginia Historical Society.

CHAPTER FOUR

1. The *Winchester Times*, "Torpedo Attack, Lieut. Glassell in Harbor at Charleston," Wednesday, June 7, 1893, p. 1.

CHAPTER FIVE

1. *SHSP*, vol. 19, pp. 93–100. This covert operation is related in the following book: Royce Gordon Shingleton, *John Taylor Wood, Sea Ghost of the Confederacy* (Athens, Ga.: The University of Georgia Press, 1979), p. 103.

2. Ralph W. Donnelly, *The Confederate States Marine Corps: The Rebel Leathernecks* (Shippensburg, Pa.: White Mane Publishing Company, Inc., 1989), p. 104.

CHAPTER SIX

1. Daniel Burr Conrad, *Blue and Gray*, vol. 4, no. 2, August 1894, pp. 92, 93.
2. *SHSP*, vol. 19, pp. 72–82.
3. Journal of James C. Palmer, fleet surgeon, from photocopy furnished by courtesy of Paul DeHaan, Kalamazoo, Michigan.
4. Document in possession of the author.
5. *SHSP*, vol. 6, p. 222.
6. Document in possession of the author.
7. Richard Curd Bowles, "The Ship 'Tennessee' and the Conflict in Mobile Bay," *Goochland County Historical Society Magazine*, vol. 26, 1994, pp. 40, 41.
8. *Naval Official Records*, ser. 1, vol. 21, p. 609.
9. Ibid, pp. 639, 640.
10. Bowles, vol. 26, 1994, pp. 35, 36
11. *Naval Official Records*, ser. 2, vol. 2, p. 758.
12. William N. Still, Jr., *Iron Afloat: The Story of the Confederate Armorclads* (Columbia, S.C.: University of South Carolina Press, 1991), pp. 225, 226.

CHAPTER SEVEN

1. Document in the possession of the author.
2. ———, *Institutional Care of the Insane*, "Central State Hospital," Chapter written by William Francis Drewry, M.D. (Baltimore, Md.: Johns Hopkins Press, 1916), pp. 733–71.
3. Richmond Civil War Centennial Committee, "Confederate Military Hospitals in Richmond," pp. 19, 20.
4. *Institutional Care of the Insane*, p. 771.
5. "Confederate Military Hospitals in Richmond," p. 19.
6. Correspondence with Ms. Catherine Roller.
7. "Confederate Military Hospitals in Richmond," p. 19.
8. Correspondence with Ms. Catherine Roller.
9. *Institutional Care of the Insane*, p. 771.
10. Blanton, p. 72.
11. Ibid., p. 167.
12. Document in the possession of the author.
13. Ibid.
14. Daniel Burr Conrad, M.D., "Some Yarns Spun by an Officer of the Old Navy," *The United Service, A Monthly Review of Military and Naval Affairs* (Philadelphia, Pa.: L. R. Hamersly & Co., vol. 8, October 1892), pp. 329, 30.
15. Document in the possession of the author.

APPENDIX

1. The *Winchester Times*, "Death of Dr. D. B. Conrad," Wednesday, September 28, 1898.

2. E. Holmes Bond, "The Conrad Boys in the Confederate Service," *Southern Historical Society Papers*, vol. 6, p. 224.

3. Ibid.

4. The *Winchester Evening Star*, "Mrs. D. B. Conrad Passes Away After a Brief Illness," Friday, September 16, 1927, p. 1.

5. Author's collection.

Bibliography

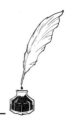

Newspapers

"Death of Dr. D. B. Conrad," The *Winchester Times*, September 28, 1898.

"Mrs. D. B. Conrad Passes Away After a Brief Illness," The *Winchester Star*, September 16, 1927.

Lazazzera, Teresa. "The True Statesman." The *Winchester Star*, November 4, 1989.

Montgomery Advertiser-Journal (Alabama), Sunday, February 19, 1961.

"'Torpedo Attack', Lieut. Glassell in Harbor at Charleston," The *Winchester Evening Times*, June 7, 1893.

The Winchester Times, January 14, 1891, printing of the monograph about the Battle of First Manassas.

The Winchester Times, August 2, 1893, begins reprint of the above monograph in two part article. (Same as in *SHSP*)

The Winchester Times, August 9, 1893, second of a two-part monograph. (Same as in *SHSP*)

The Winchester Times, September 21, 1898, announcement of Dr. Conrad's death but more complete obituary provided in the following week's edition.

The Winchester Times, September 28, 1898, full obituary of Dr. Daniel Burr Conrad.

Periodicals

Blue and Gray Magazine. The Current Publishing Company, Philadelphia, Pa. January 1895 and September 1894.

Bowles, Richard Curd. *Goochland County Historical Society Magazine*, vol. 26, 1994.

Conrad, Daniel Burr. *The United Service, A Monthly Review of Military and Naval Affairs,* "Some Yarns Spun By an Officer of the Old Navy," vol. 8, October 1892.

List of Officers of the Navy of the United States and of the Marine Corps, New York, 1901.

Riggs, David F. *The Virginia Magazine of History and Biography,* vol. 86, July 1978.

Rutherford, Phillip. "The New Bern Raid." *Civil War Times,* January 1982.

Southern Historical Society Papers, 6, pp. 220-27.

Southern Historical Society Papers, 21, pp. 290-94.

Southern Historical Society Papers, 30, p. 232.

Southern Historical Society Papers, 19, pp. 93-100.

Southern Historical Society Papers, 19, pp. 72-82.

United States Army and Navy Magazine. Conrad's obituary said he wrote some article in this magazine, [unable to locate].

Books

——. *Institutional Care of the Insane,* "Central State Hospital." Chapter written by William Francis Drewry, M.D. Baltimore, Md.: Johns Hopkins Press, 1916, pp. 733-71.

Amadon, George F. *Rise of the Ironclads.* Missoula, Mont.: Pictorial Histories Publishing Company, 1995.

Campbell, R. Thomas. *Southern Thunder: Exploits of the Confederate States Navy.* Shippensburg, Pa.: Burd Street Press, 1997.

Coski, John M. *Capital Navy.* Campbell, Calif.: Savas Woodbury Publishers, 1996.

Cunningham, H. H. *Doctors in Gray.* Gloucester, Mass.: Louisiana State University Press, 1970.

Donnelly, Ralph W. *The Confederate States Marine Corps: The Rebel Leathernecks.* Shippensburg, Pa.: White Mane Publishing Company, Inc., 1989.

Frye, Dennis E. *2nd Virginia Infantry.* Lynchburg, Va.: H. E. Howard, Inc., 1984.

Hearn, Chester G. *Mobile Bay and the Mobile Campaign.* Jefferson, N.C.: McFarland Company, Inc., 1993.

Hoehling, A. A. *Damn The Torpedoes! Naval Incidents of the Civil War.* Winston-Salem, N.C.: John F. Blair, publisher, 1989.

Lewis, Charles Lee. *Admiral Franklin Buchanan, Fearless Man of Action.* Baltimore, Md.: The Norman Remington Company, 1929.

Luraghi, Raimondo. *A History of the Confederate Navy.* Annapolis, Md.: Naval Institute Press, 1996.

Mokin, Arthur. *Ironclad: The Monitor & the Merrimack.* Novato, Calif.: Presidio Press, 1991.

Musicant, Ivan. *Divided Waters: The Naval History of the Civil War.* New York, N.Y.: Harper Collins Publishers, 1995.

Naval History Division, Navy Department. *Civil War Naval Chronology, 1861-1865.* Washington, D.C.: 1971.

Official Records of the Union and Confederate Navies, ser. 1, vol. 21, and ser. 2, vols. 1 and 2. Washington, D.C.: Government Printing Office.

Pratt, Fletcher. *The Compact History of the United States Navy.* New York: Hawthorn Books, Inc., 1967.

Quarles, Garland R. *The Story of One Hundred Old Homes in Winchester, Virginia,* 1993.

Rich, Doris. *Fort Morgan.* Foley, Ala.: Underwood Printing Co., 1986.

Rye, Scott. *Men and Ships of the Civil War.* Stamford, Conn.: Longmeadow Press, 1995.

Schildt, John W. *Hunter Holmes McGuire, Doctor in Gray.* Chewsville, Md.: 1986.

Shingleton, Royce Gordon. *John Taylor Wood, Sea Ghost of the Confederacy.* Athens, Ga.: The University of Georgia Press, 1979.

Shomette, Donald G. *Shipwrecks of the Civil War.* Washington, D.C.: Donic Ltd., 1973.

Silverstone, Paul H. *Warships of the Civil War Navies.* Annapolis, Md.: Naval Institute Press, 1989.

Stern, Philip Van Doren. *The Confederate Navy.* New York, N.Y.: Bonanza Books, 1962.

Still, William N., Jr. *Iron Afloat, The Story of the Confederate Armorclads.* Columbia, S.C.: University of South Carolina Press, 1991.

Still, William N., Jr. *Odyssey in Gray.* Richmond, Va.: Virginia State Library, 1979.

Still, William N,. Jr. Ed. *Odyssey in Gray: A Diary of Confederate Service, Douglas French Forrest.* Richmond, Va.: Virginia State Library, 1979.

The United Service, A Monthly Review of Military and Naval Affairs. Philadelphia, Pa.: L. R. Hamersly & Co., October 1892.

Logs found at the National Archives of ships with which Conrad was affiliated: *Congress, Plymouth, Niagara, Savannah, Saranac, Susquehanna, and Tennessee.*

Correspondence

Central State Hospital, Archives, Petersburg, Virginia.

Chicago Historical Society, Chicago, Illinois.

Eastern State Hospital, Archives, Williamsburg, Virginia.

Handley Regional Library, Winchester, Virginia.

The Mariner's Museum, Newport News, Virginia.

Museum of the Confederacy, Richmond, Virginia.

The Naval Historical Center, Washington, D.C.

Tulane University, Howard-Tilton Memorial Library, New Orleans, Louisiana.

University of Pennsylvania, The University Archives and Records Center, North Arcade, Franklin Field, Philadelphia, Pennsylvania.

University of Virginia Library, Special Collections Department, Alderman Library, Charlottesville, Virginia.

Virginia Commonwealth University, Medical College of Virginia, Thompkins-McCaw Library, Archives.

Virginia Historical Society, Richmond, Virginia.

Virginia State Library, Richmond, Virginia.

Western State Hospital, Archives, Staunton, Virginia.

Winchester-Frederick County Historical Society, Winchester, Virginia.

Index

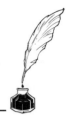

Spezia, Italy, 14
Springfield, Massachusetts, 181
Staunton, Virginia, 96, 167, 171, 177, 179
Stephens City, Virginia, 168, 182
Strait of Gibraltar, 14

T

Tattnall, Com. Josiah, 40
Tomb, Asst. Eng. James H., 111
Toulon, France, 14, 19, 20, 24
Tredegar Iron Works, 42

U

United Service (periodical), 174
University of Pennsylvania, Philadelphia, Pennsylvania, 5, 173, 182-83
University of Virginia, Charlottesville, Virginia, 2, 33, 82, 176, 178, 179, 182
USS *Chickasaw*, 152, 155
USS *Colorado*, 30
USS *Congress*, 8, 11, 14, 16, 20, 25, 152, 177
USS *Constellation*, 8, 30, 52, 53
USS *Hartford*, 139, 145, 149, 152, 155, 156-57, 159, 163-64
USS *Monitor*, 8, 136
USS *Monongahela*, 155
USS *Montauk*, 87
USS *Nashville*, 86
USS *New Ironsides*, 111, 112, 116
USS *Niagara*, 1, 39, 40, 62
USS *North Carolina*, 61
USS *Pawnee*, 46
USS *Plymouth*, 30, 32
USS *Powhatan*, 40, 42
USS *Saganaw*, 56, 57
USS *San Jacinto*, 8, 52, 53
USS *Saranac*, 8
USS *Savannah* (steamer), 18, 20, 35
USS *Tuscarora*, 86
USS *Underwriter*, 2, 117-18, 125, 129, 174, 177

V

Valley of Jehoshaphat, 25
Virginia Military Institute (VMI), Lexington, Virginia, 12, 64
Virginia navy, 1, 64

W

Western State Hospital, 171, 177
Wheat, Maj. Chatham Roberdeau, 79
Winchester *Evening Star*, 180
Winchester Medical College, Winchester, Virginia, 2, 4, 176
Winchester *Times*, 111, 173
Winchester, Virginia, 1, 2, 6, 18, 24, 30, 33, 35, 61, 62, 63, 66-67, 69, 70, 94-96, 97, 98, 101, 103-4, 106, 109, 110, 111, 167, 168, 173, 175, 176, 178, 179, 180, 181, 183, 184
Wood, Comdr. John Taylor, 2, 117, 118-19, 121, 123, 129
Worden, Comdr. John, 87